GET OFF THE DIET-GO-ROUND. GET ON WITH YOUR LIFE.

START WHERE YOU ARE WEIGHT LOSS

PLAYBOOK

SHELLI JOHNSON

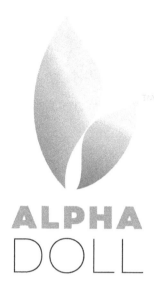

START WHERE YOU ARE WEIGHT LOSS PLAYBOOK

For information:
startwhereyouareweightloss.com

Also available now!

SELF-HELP BOOKS

Start Where You Are Weight Loss
Start Where You Are Weight Loss Manifesto
Start Where You Are Weight Loss Freedom Commandments
Baby Step Your Way to a Life You Love: Encourage Yourself
Baby Step Your Way to a Life You Love: Forgive Yourself
Baby Step Your Way to a Life You Love: Heal Your Burned-Out Self
Baby Step Your Way to a Life You Love: Overcome Fear
Baby Step Your Way to a Life You Love: Crush Self-Doubt
Baby Step Your Way to a Life You Love: Get Out of Your Own Way
Baby Step Your Way to a Life You Love: Become Yourself
Baby Step Your Way to a Life You Love: Let Go

ADULT COLORING BOOKS

Color Your Way to a Life You Love: Encourage Yourself
Color Your Way to a Life You Love: Forgive Yourself
Color Your Way to a Life You Love: Heal Your Burned-Out Self
Color Your Way to a Life You Love: Overcome Fear
Color Your Way to a Life You Love: Crush Self-Doubt
Color Your Way to a Life You Love: Get Out of Your Own Way
Color Your Way to a Life You Love: Become Yourself
Color Your Way to a Life You Love: Let Go

NOVELS

Small as a Mustard Seed

CHILDREN'S BOOKS

Leave Me Alone

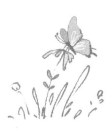

Contents!

This is a companion book!

COMPANION TO START WHERE YOU ARE WEIGHT LOSS

This book was designed to give you the opportunity to answer probing questions, explore your innermost thoughts and feelings, chart your progress and successes, along with other encouraging activities, all in one convenient place. Complete instructions and explanations for this book can be found in its companion book:
Start Where You Are Weight Loss (ISBN: 978-1-948103-81-7)

Don't scare yourself!

DON'T OVERWHELM YOURSELF EITHER

I know this book looks intimidating by its sheer size. Don't be scared. Don't be overwhelmed. Don't let any anxiety rise in you about how you're going to make it through or how much work (play!) it may be or anything else regarding this book that you may be anxious about right now.

This book is meant to be done slowly over the length of your weight-loss journey. It's going to take some time to get to where you want to be. Take that time to learn some things about yourself in this playbook. Learn what you really need, what you honestly want, what deeply matters to you. Learn why you abuse food. Learn what you need to do to best take care of yourself so that you can stop the food-abuse cycle and move forward in a straight line to create a body and a life that you love. You have permission, always, to go as slowly as you need to go so that you don't scare and/or overwhelm yourself

Every day, you just take a deep breath and start where you are.

Visual reminders!

BUTTERFLIES AND WORDS

The butterflies in this book are there to remind you that you're on a journey to transform yourself and your life. If you'll just keep going, you will experience a transformation. The decorative words scattered throughout are ones you can use to describe yourself and speak strength to yourself.

A few helpful suggestions!

BABY STEPS

I'm a big believer in the power of taking baby steps to get you anywhere you need or want to go, which is why this book is written the way it is. Each small-sized activity builds on another, one to the next. So just know you'll be best served to do the activities in order.

NO PERFECTION NEEDED

Do yourself a kindness and make a mistake in this playbook early on. Scribble on some of the pages. Spill your favorite beverage on the cover. Rip one of the corners off. Make this book imperfect so that you'll feel free to be your real, honest self inside the pages. Being real, not being perfect, is what's going to heal you and set you free.

BE HONEST

I'd recommend that you don't show your answers inside this playbook to anyone. Keep them to yourself for right now until you make it all the way through to the end. Why? Honesty with yourself is what's going to help you heal and grow. You won't be completely honest if you're worried about someone reading your answers. In fact, what you're likely to do is tweak your responses, edit them, or scratch them out entirely if you're worried about how others might perceive you. So be kind to yourself & let this playbook be just for you.

BE WILLING & OPEN

The first step to change is to be open & willing to it. You picked up this playbook because you're struggling in this area of your life. If you want things to be different, well, both you & those things are going to have to change. So be open to experiencing something new & be willing to do the effort to get there.

GIVE YOURSELF PERMISSION

It's hugely important to give yourself permission (whether that's verbally or written) to: do the suggestions in this playbook, be/have/do/say/believe whatever you need to so that you can heal yourself, give yourself unlimited tries as many times as it takes, believe in your own worth and value, choose to create a life you love because you matter. Whenever you feel like you need someone else's permission to make a choice about your life, you just give that permission to yourself. The only permission you ever need to live your own life is your own.

YOU'RE ON A JOURNEY

It doesn't matter how old you are, how many times you've tried, or how far there is left to go. It's never too late to be the person you want to be. It's okay if you don't know things yet. You're on a journey and you'll figure it out as you go. This playbook is designed to help you do just that.

BEGIN YOUR DAY WITH A STEP

If at all possible, read a little (don't overwhelm yourself) of the companion book (Start Where You Are daily then do the corresponding suggestion shortly after you wake up. That way, you'll be able to focus on yourself (because you're absolutely worth the time to do that) before your day gets away from you. Find a quiet place. Relax and reflect.

IT'S A PRACTICE & A PROCESS

There's no doing this perfectly, and that's okay. You strive for progress. You do the best you can. So show yourself some patience and kindness because self-compassion is what you most need to heal yourself. You will make mistakes, there's just no way around it. Don't ever use any mistake as a reason to give up on yourself. Just circle back around and start again. And know this: every mistake is simply a brand new chance to do it better the next time.

AND FINALLY . . .

Remember (not just for this book but for all of life): you get out what you put in. So make yourself a priority in your own life because: 1. you're absolutely worth the effort and 2. no one else can do it for you. And one last suggestion good both for this book and for all of life: be brave and move beyond your fear, that's where freedom lies.

Cherry pick!

ANSWER WHAT RESONATES WITH YOU

Both Start Where You Are Weight Loss and this companion book were written to address the concerns/issues that I encountered during my weight-loss journey and the steps I took to find freedom from being overweight and from abusing food. It's entirely possible that you will not have exactly the same concerns/issues/experiences during your own journey to freedom. So some of the questions and/or activities in this book may not apply to you. Feel free, always, to respond to those questions/activities that resonate with your particular situation and skip those that don't. Make this playbook your own.

Be brave!

Life don't often ask your permission first, that's true.
And sometimes you find yourself wandering
around in the dark.

It's real likely that you might stumble across
somebody else's path out there in the dimness.
You might even follow it for a time, trying
to get your bearings, and that's okay.

But in the end, you got find your own path in this world.
Ain't nobody that can do it for you.

Because if you keep on following in somebody else's footsteps,
you ain't ever gonna learn who you are,
you ain't ever gonna learn who you could become.

—Ned Horner

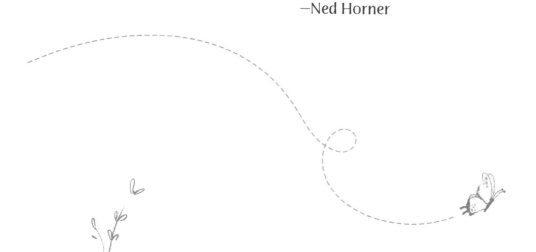

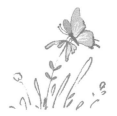

Those who are brave are free!

"It is not the critic who counts; not the man who points out how the strong man stumbles, or where the doer of deeds could have done them better. The credit belongs to the man who is actually in the arena, whose face is marred by dust and sweat and blood; who strives valiantly; who errs, who comes short again and again, because there is no effort without error and shortcoming; but who does actually strive to do the deeds; who knows great enthusiasms, the great devotions; who spends himself in a worthy cause; who at the best knows in the end the triumph of high achievement, and who at the worst, if he fails, at least fails while daring greatly, so that his place shall never be with those cold and timid souls who neither know victory nor defeat."

—Theodore Roosevelt

Source: excerpt (also known as "The Man In The Arena") from the speech "Citizenship in a Republic" delivered at The Sorbonne in Paris, France on April 23, 1910.

"The meaning of life is to find your gift. The purpose of life is to give it away."

—Pablo Picasso

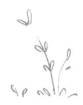

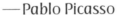

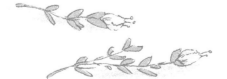

Preface!

♡ What does being thin mean/symbolize for you? ♡

_____

_____

_____

♡ Write a list of things you've tried to lose weight (no matter how detrimental to your well-being)? ♡

_____

_____

_____

_____

_____

♡ Write down five things that are awesome about you. ♡

1. _____

2. _____

3. _____

4. _____

5. _____

♡ Read that list aloud. ♡

⌒ If your courage was bigger than your fear — and don't worry, soon it will be —
what would you most want to dare to do with your life? ⌒

_____

_____

_____

_____

_____

⌒ Oh yes, you can! ⌒

⌒ What do you think your purpose is? (It's okay if you don't know, just write down
what you think it might be.) ⌒

_____

_____

_____

_____

_____

⌒ Are you happy with the path you're on right now? If not, what path would you
rather be on? ⌒

_____

_____

❧ **Who do you think you are? Who do you want to become?** ☙

_____

_____

_____

_____

_____

_____

_____

❧ Remember: the only person you are destined to be is the person you decide to become. ☙
❧ (Quote from Ralph Waldo Emerson) ☙

❧ **What would you be doing with your life, right now, if you weren't so focused on being stuck on the diet-go-round?** ☙

_____

_____

_____

_____

_____

_____

_____

_____

What are you waiting for permission from others to have/be/do/say before you will step out and have/be/do/say those things?

_____

_____

_____

_____

_____

_____

_____

_____

Remember: all that waiting is all that time you can never get back.

Use the space below to write a permission slip to yourself to have/be/do/say what you most want.

Then sign your name and date.

_____

_____

_____

_____

_____

_____

Name:_____**Date:**_____

Honor yourself and keep your word to yourself.

Love Yourself!

♡ Write an instance when you were shamed/humiliated because of your weight. ♡

_____

_____

_____

♡ Now take a deep breath, hold three seconds, then let it slowly out of your mouth. ♡

♡ Now write ten things you admire or appreciate about yourself. ♡

1. _____

2. _____

3. _____

4. _____

5. _____

6. _____

7. _____

8. _____

9. _____

10. _____

♡ Read that list aloud. ♡

♡ Write an instance when you turned to food for comfort. ♡

_____

_____

_____

♡ Now write an instance when you showed strength and courage when no food was involved. ♡

_____

_____

_____

♡ Write an instance when you have harmed your body or mind in an attempt to lose weight. ♡

_____

_____

_____

♡ Now write one thing you most need to do to heal yourself that has nothing to do with food/eating. ♡

_____

_____

_____

♡ Go do that thing today, guilt-free. ♡

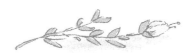

♡ Write an instance when you lost hope. ♡

_____

_____

_____

♡ Now write an instance for which you still harbor a sprig of hope. ♡

_____

_____

_____

♡ Write an instance when you hated your body or part of your body. ♡

_____

_____

_____

♡ Now take a deep breath, hold three seconds, then let it slowly out of your mouth. ♡

♡ Now write an instance when you loved your body and what it could do and/or let you feel.

_____

_____

_____

♡ Pause. Let that time you loved your body really sink in. ♡

⌒ Then write five things that you are grateful to your body for. ⌒

1. _____

2. _____

3. _____

4. _____

5. _____

⌒ Read that list aloud. ⌒

⌒ Write an instance when you felt ugly. ⌒

_____

_____

_____

⌒ Now take a deep breath, hold three seconds, then let it slowly out of your mouth. ⌒

⌒ Now write an instance when you felt beautiful. ⌒

_____

_____

_____

⌒ Pause. Let that time you felt beautiful really sink in. ⌒

◁ Write an instance when you showed weakness. ▷

_____

_____

_____

◁ Now write an instance when you were stronger than you thought yourself ever capable of being. ▷

_____

_____

_____

◁ Write an instance when you lied to yourself. ▷

_____

_____

_____

◁ Now write an instance when you told yourself the absolute truth and let the chips fall where they would. ▷

_____

_____

_____

_____

❧ Write an instance when you beat yourself up for something you did or something you failed to do. ☙

_____

_____

_____

❧ Now write an instance when you practiced self-compassion and forgave yourself for your mistakes. ☙

_____

_____

_____

❧ Remember: self-compassion is what you most need to heal yourself. ☙

❧ Write an instance when you quit. ☙

_____

_____

_____

❧ Now write an instance when you kept going and refused to give up. ☙

_____

_____

_____

♡ Write an instance when you felt stupid. ♡

_____

_____

_____

♡ Now write an instance when you proved to yourself just how intelligent you really are. ♡

_____

_____

_____

♡ Write an instance when you waited for someone to come save/fix your life. ♡

_____

_____

_____

♡ Now write an instance when you saved/fixed your own life. ♡

_____

_____

_____

Some Guidance for the Journey!

·» Your time on the diet-go-round «·

ᴕ Write your age now: ᴕ _____

ᴕ Write your age when you started dieting: ᴕ _____

ᴕ Subtract: ᴕ _____

ᴕ That's how long you've been on the diet-go-round. ᴕ
ᴕ Now take a deep breath, hold three seconds, then let it slowly out of your mouth. ᴕ

ᴕ Answer this honestly: Do you want to keep spinning on the diet-go-round or would you like to jump off? ᴕ _____

·» Listen for your voice of wisdom «·

ᴕ Are you willing to believe that your intuition is there to encourage you, strengthen you, guide you, and help you grow? Are you willing to believe that your intuition will never tear you down or berate you? Why or why not? ᴕ

_____

_____

_____

ᴕ Do you believe all the answers you need to fix your life truly are inside of you? Why or why not? ᴕ

_____

_____

_____

◁ Do you trust yourself? Why or why not? ▷

_____

_____

_____

◁ Know this: self-trust is paramount to your success. ▷

◁ Write some questions about your life that you'd like the answers to. ▷

_____

_____

_____

_____

_____

_____

_____

_____

_____

_____

_____

꒰ Look inward for guidance. Be open (so no overthinking and/or editing). Write the answers that come. ꒱

_____

_____

_____

_____

_____

_____

_____

_____

_____

_____

_____

_____

_____

_____

_____

_____

_____

_____

❧ Write down the names of any other people's voices clamoring for your attention. Will you listen to them or to yourself? ❧

_____

_____

_____

_____

_____

_____

_____

_____

❧ Will you do what your intuition tells you to do? Why or why not? ❧

_____

_____

_____

❧ Are you willing to be completely honest with yourself? Why or why not? ❧

_____

_____

_____

·» Answer a single question «·

♡ The wound is the something(s) that you feel/think/believe is (or are) lacking in you. Listen for your intuition and answer this: What is that wound for you? ♡

_____

_____

_____

_____

_____

_____

♡ Remember: the wound is the place where the light enters you. ♡
♡ (Quote from Jalaluddin Rumi) ♡

♡ Do you believe you are broken? If so, why? ♡

_____

_____

_____

_____

_____

♡ Now take a deep breath, hold three seconds, then let it slowly out of your mouth. ♡

⊘ If you believe you are broken, what do you think you need to do to fix yourself? Or do you believe that you are not fixable? ⋄

_____

_____

_____

_____

⊘ Are you willing to believe there is nothing broken in you, that you are whole (something that is complete in itself) already, right now, just the way you are? Why or why not? ⋄

_____

_____

_____

·⁀ Always give yourself permission «·

⊘ Use the space below to write a permission slip to yourself for anything else you want for your life not mentioned earlier (on page 13). ⋄
⊘ Then sign your name and date. ⋄

_____

_____

_____

_____

_____

Name:_____**Date:**_____
⊘ Oh yes, you can! ⋄

·» The freedom commandments «·

◌ Write each of these in your own handwriting then say them out loud: ◌

◌ I will let go, right now, of doing any of this perfectly. ◌

_____

◌ I will take the pressure off and cut myself some slack and not beat myself up. ◌

_____

_____

◌ I will not measure my self-worth by how much I weigh, how many mistakes I make, how much money I earn, how many friends I have, and any other transient measurement. ◌

_____

_____

_____

_____

◌ I will start believing in myself and believing in possibility. ◌

_____

_____

◌ I will stop listening to what everyone else tells me that I should do and start listening to my own intuition. ◌

_____

_____

_____

♡ I will stop waiting for my life to begin when I weigh a certain amount and/or wear a certain size and instead I will start enjoying my life today. ♡

_____

_____

_____

♡ I will be kind, gentle, and patient with myself. ♡

_____

♡ I will not compare myself and my life to anyone else's. ♡

_____

♡ I will take excellent care of myself and put myself at the top of my to-do list. ♡

_____

_____

♡ I will forgive myself for my mistakes and failures. ♡

_____

♡ I will stop judging and labeling myself. ♡

_____

♡ I will realize that I can't ever go back, so I will go forward instead. ♡

_____

_____

♡ I will not act on how I feel at the moment but on what I know to be true. ♡

_____

_____

❧ I will put my blinders on and take the next right step and stop looking at the obstacles to overcome and the reasons why not. ❧

_____

_____

_____

❧ I will not give up. ❧

_____

·» You are enough as-is «·

❧ Write this five times: I am enough as-is. ❧

1. _____

2. _____

3. _____

4. _____

5. _____

❧ Look yourself in the eyes in a mirror. Say that to yourself five times. ❧

❧ Do you believe you are enough as-is, right now, as you are? Why or why not? ❧

_____

_____

_____

_____

♡ If you don't believe you are enough as-is, are you open and willing to believe it? Why or why not? ♡

_____

_____

_____

♡ Write this five times again: I am enough as-is. ♡

1. _____

2. _____

3. _____

4. _____

5. _____

♡ Look yourself in the eyes in a mirror. Say that to yourself five times. ♡

·» There may be some pain «·

♡ Will you sit with yourself and let yourself feel the pain? Why or why not? ♡

_____

_____

_____

♡ Write an instance when something bad happened to you that you just didn't understand at the time. ♡

_____

_____

_____

♡ Now write how that bad thing turned out to be a gift (learned a lesson, opened a different path in your life, brought you new relationships, etc.) and worked out for your good. ♡

_____

_____

_____

_____

♡ Now encourage yourself and write kind words that you most need to hear right now to reassure yourself. ♡

_____

_____

_____

_____

♡ Look yourself in the eyes in a mirror then read those words aloud. ♡

·» Listen to your own self and your own body «·

⊘ Do you believe you're powerless? Why or why not? ⊘

_____

_____

_____

⊘ Do you believe you have no choices? Why or why not? ⊘

_____

_____

_____

⊘ What do you believe about food and its role in your life? ⊘

_____

_____

_____

_____

_____

_____

_____

_____

◌ What do you believe about the current state of your life? ◌

_____

_____

_____

_____

_____

◌ Do you believe you are capable of changing what you believe and changing your life? Why or why not? ◌

_____

_____

_____

·» Cherry pick «·

◌ Write a list of diets and/or food plans you've been on. ◌

_____

_____

_____

_____

_____

♡ Write anything that worked for you &/or that you enjoyed about those particular diets and/or food plans. ♡

_____

_____

_____

_____

_____

_____

_____

_____

_____

_____

_____

_____

_____

_____

_____

_____

_____

_____

♡ Combining anything that worked for you &/or things you enjoyed, what would the ideal diet/food plan/way of eating/lifestyle look like to you? ♡

·» Take these to heart «·

♡ Write this three times: Food is fuel for my body. ♡

1. _____

2. _____

3. _____

♡ Write this three times: Food will not fix it. ♡

1. _____

2. _____

3. _____

♡ Write this three times: No one is coming. ♡

1. _____

2. _____

3. _____

♡ Write this three times: I must trust myself. ♡

1. _____

2. _____

3. _____

♡ Look yourself in the eyes in a mirror. Say each of those to yourself three times. ♡

◁ Write this three times: I must save myself. ▷

1. _____

2. _____

3. _____

◁ Look yourself in the eyes in a mirror. Say that to yourself three times. ▷

⟫ Give yourself a prize ⟪

◁ Write a list of prizes (nonfood items) that you would love to receive. ▷

_____

_____

_____

_____

_____

_____

_____

_____

_____

_____

◁ Now assign a goal to each. When you reach that goal, you get that prize. ▷

◁ Build self-trust and honor your word. Be sure to give yourself that prize. ▷

Chapter One!

•» Some things to consider before you even get started «•

•» Check your motivation «•

♡ For whom are you losing weight and/or stopping food abuse? For you or for someone else? If it's for someone else, write their name(s). ♡

_____

_____

♡ Whether it's for you or for someone else, why do you want to lose weight and/or stop abusing food? ♡

_____

_____

_____

_____

♡ Do you believe that you, yourself, are a rock-solid foundation for your life that you can count on? Why or why not? ♡

_____

_____

_____

♡ Remember: self-trust is paramount to your success. ♡

⌁ Do you believe you are strong, courageous, gifted, talented, amazing, worthwhile, and completely capable of shedding the weight and/or of not abusing food so you can live the life you want? Why or why not? ⌁

_____

_____

_____

_____

⌁ Does being comfortable in your own body matter deeply to you? If not, why not? ⌁

_____

_____

_____

⌁ Do you believe you're worth the effort? Why or why not? ⌁

_____

_____

_____

⌁ You are worth the effort. ⌁

⌁ Will you choose to lose weight for you and you alone? Why or why not? ⌁

_____

_____

_____

›› Blame will not help you ‹‹

◌ Who or what, if anyone or anything, are you blaming for your weight, your current predicaments, and/or the way your life turned out? Why? ◌

_____

_____

_____

_____

_____

_____

_____

◌ What will you do if they never admit to what they did? What will you do if they never make amends? What will you do if they never come to fix what's wrong? ◌

_____

_____

_____

_____

_____

_____

_____

◌ Remember: the only way to get your power back is to take it. So take it back. ◌

❤ Do you believe you are one-hundred-percent responsible for what you eat and how much you weigh? Why or why not? ❤

_____

_____

_____

❤ Do you believe you are fully responsible for your own life, your own choices, and how your life turns out? Why or why not? ❤

_____

_____

_____

❤ Do you believe you are the boss of you? Why or why not? ❤

_____

_____

_____

❤ What characteristics would your ideal boss have? ❤

_____

_____

_____

_____

⊰ Are you willing to be an ideal boss to yourself? Why or why not? ⊱

_____

_____

_____

⊰ What lesson(s) can you learn from the people/things you are blaming? ⊱

_____

_____

_____

_____

_____

_____

_____

_____

⊰ Are you willing to stop blaming other people/things and take your power back? Why or why not? ⊱

_____

_____

_____

⊰ Remember: the only way to get your power back is to take it. So take it back. ⊱

·» Self-pity is a sheer cliff into a black abyss «·

♡ Are you feeling sorry for yourself at the moment? If so, why? ♥

_____

_____

_____

_____

♡ Do you BELIEVE you can get yourself out of the mess you've made (with your weight or with your life)? Why or why not? ♥

_____

_____

_____

♡ Do you WANT to get yourself out of the mess you've made (with your weight or with your life)? Why or why not? ♥

_____

_____

_____

♡ Are you willing to take action, make a plan, and take steps forward to get yourself where you want to be? Why or why not? ♥

_____

_____

_____

·» You'll have to interrupt the pattern so you can grow «·

◁ What patterns do you see yourself doing in your life? ▷

_____

_____

_____

_____

_____

_____

_____

◁ Are you willing to change? Why or why not? ▷

_____

_____

_____

◁ Know this: change really is your friend. ▷

◁ Are you open to doing things differently and seeing your life in a new light? Why or why not? ▷

_____

_____

_____

◁ Imagine how powerful you'd be if you'd simply interrupt the pattern. ▷

Are you willing to be okay with uncertainty and relax into the space between where you are now and where you most want to be? Why or why not?

_____

_____

_____

Just be open to the possibility of doing things differently.

How will you let that in-between space motivate you instead of scare you?

_____

_____

_____

_____

_____

_____

_____

Just be willing and open.

Are you willing to let yourself be a beginner again? Why or why not?

_____

_____

_____

·» It's likely going to take longer than you think «·

♡ How long are you hoping it will take to reach your weight-loss goal? ♡

_____

♡ Are you willing to accept, right now, that your weight loss may take longer (even a lot longer) to achieve? Why or why not? ♡

_____

_____

_____

♡ Do you understand that you're in your body until your life is over, regardless of whether you're at peace with your body or not? ♡ _____

♡ Are you willing to have patience, keep going, and not give up on yourself regardless of how long it takes for you to reach your goal(s)? Why or why not? ♡

_____

_____

_____

♡ Know this: patience really is your friend. ♡

·» Some lies you'll have to stop believing «·

♡ Listen for your intuition, be honest with yourself, and write your own list of lies you need to stop believing. ♡

_____

_____

_____

_____

_____

_____

_____

_____

_____

_____

_____

_____

_____

♡ Read over that list. Add any lies that you may have forgotten. ♡

♡ Now write a mantra to directly combat that lie, which you'll repeat to yourself and believe instead. ♡

♡ Read that list aloud. ♡

» Lie: Losing/Maintaining weight loss is hard and gets harder with age and/or nothing is harder than breaking food abuse «

◊ What do you believe about losing weight and maintaining weight loss? ◊

_____

_____

_____

_____

_____

_____

_____

◊ What do you believe about breaking food abuse? ◊

_____

_____

_____

_____

_____

_____

_____

◊ Remember: you will always live out what you believe. So choose beliefs that will help you. ◊

·» Lie: You have to live this way «·

⊲ What do you believe about being stuck living the way you are living? ⊳

_____

_____

_____

_____

_____

_____

_____

⊲ Remember: your beliefs are not by chance, they are by choice. So choose differently. ⊳

·» Lie: You are not worth the effort and/or you don't have what it takes «·

⊲ What do you believe about your own worth and value? ⊳

_____

_____

_____

_____

_____

_____

⊲ Remember: you will always live out what you believe. ⊳

◌ Are you willing, right now and always, to treat yourself with kindness and respect? Why or why not? ◌

_____

_____

_____

◌ Remember: you have worth and value because you are alive. ◌

Are you willing to treat yourself, always, as the worthy and valuable person you are? Why or why not? ◌

_____

_____

_____

◌ Remember: you have everything inside you to create a life you love. ◌

◌ Write five nice things you could do to take excellent care of yourself. ◌

1. _____

2. _____

3. _____

4. _____

5. _____

◌ Do one (or more!) today. ◌

♡ Write a list of all your accomplishments (no matter how big or small). ♡

_____

_____

_____

_____

_____

_____

_____

_____

_____

_____

_____

_____

_____

_____

_____

_____

♡ Reread that list often. Add to it as you accomplish more things. ♡

·» Lie: Loneliness will break you «·

♡ What do you believe about feelings being able to break you? ♡

_____

_____

_____

_____

_____

_____

_____

♡ Remember: a feeling only has the power that you give it and feelings pass. ♡
♡ Remember: you are whole as you are. ♡

·» Lie: Your life is not your own and/or your life is a dress rehearsal «·

♡ What do you believe about who/what has authority over your life? ♡

_____

_____

_____

_____

_____

♡ Remember: you're the only one responsible for your happiness. ♡

❧ What do you believe about your life happening now and putting it hold? ☙

_____

_____

_____

_____

_____

_____

❧ Remember: all the time spent waiting is all the time you can never get back. ☙

❧ Are you willing to believe that abusing food is putting your life on hold? Why or why not? ☙

_____

_____

_____

❧ Write a list of instances where you said no when you really wanted to say yes. ☙

_____

_____

_____

_____

_____

❧ Why are you putting your life on hold? ❧

_____

_____

_____

_____

❧ What do you hope to gain by waiting? ❧

_____

_____

_____

_____

❧ Who will you upset by claiming authority over your own life? ❧

_____

_____

_____

_____

❧ What are you afraid will happen if you move forward? ❧

_____

_____

_____

_____

᪣ Are you willing to take action today and move forward through that fear? Why or why not? ᪣

_____

_____

_____

᪣ Remember: your life belongs to you and you alone, you get to choose how you want to live it. ᪣
᪣ Remember: you are responsible for saving your own life. ᪣

·» Lie: You're being selfish «·

᪣ What do you believe about making yourself a priority in your own life? ᪣

_____

_____

_____

_____

_____

_____

_____

᪣ Remember: taking excellent care of yourself is the healthiest thing you can do. ᪣

❧ Write your to-do list then put your name at the top of that list. ☙

_____

_____

_____

_____

_____

_____

❧ Go do something nice for you today. ☙

·❱❱ Lie: This is who you are (and always will be) ❰❰·

❧ What do you believe about what others have said about you and who you are? ☙

_____

_____

_____

_____

_____

_____

❧ Remember: you are who you believe you are. ☙
❧ Remember: the only person you are is the one you decide to be. ☙
❧ Remember: the only opinion that matters about your life is your own. ☙

·» Lie: You are damaged goods «·

◁ What do you believe about being damaged goods or broken beyond repair? ▷

_____

_____

_____

_____

_____

_____

◁ Remember: the essence of who you are, who you are deep down, is healthy and whole. ▷

·» Lie: You don't belong unless you're someone else «·

◁ What do you believe about being someone else just so you can belong? ▷

_____

_____

_____

_____

_____

◁ Remember: the only way to free yourself is to be yourself. ▷

·» Lie: You cannot control what you think/believe «·

♡ What do you believe about being able to accept or reject negative thoughts and beliefs? ♡

_____

_____

_____

_____

_____

_____

♡ Have you ever used negative thoughts/beliefs as a distraction? If so, what are you trying to avoid? ♡

_____

_____

_____

_____

_____

_____

_____

❀ Write a list of thoughts/beliefs that you continually repeat to yourself and/or ones that are holding you back. ❀

_____

_____

_____

_____

_____

_____

_____

_____

_____

_____

_____

_____

_____

❀ Now for each thought/belief ask: Is this thought/belief honestly true? ❀

❀ Then ask: Does it serve me? ❀

❀ Then ask: Is it helping me or harming me to think/believe this? ❀

❀ Remember: you get to accept or reject any thought/belief that pops into your mind. ❀

❀ Remember: all you have to do to change your life is change your mind. ❀

·» Some things you'll have to start doing «·

·» Tell the truth «·

♡ Are you willing to always tell the honest-to-goodness truth about how you really think and feel to others, and more importantly, to yourself? Why or why not? ♡

_____

_____

_____

♡ Write a list of lies you have told and/or continue to tell to yourself and/or others. Be honest with yourself. ♡

_____

_____

_____

_____

_____

_____

_____

_____

_____

♡ Write a list of truths that you need to admit/say. Be honest with yourself. ♡

♡ Find your voice, stand up for yourself, speak those truths, and let the chips fall where they may. ♡
♡ You have it in you. Oh yes, you do. ♡
♡ You are strong, courageous, tenacious, and determined to fix your own life. Oh yes, you are. ♡

·» Make weight loss a journey you're on by yourself «·

♡ Are you willing to make weight loss and/or the cessation of abusing food a journey you're on by yourself? Why or why not? ♡

_____

_____

_____

♡ How can you make the journey more of a stroll up a hill instead of a trek up a mountain? ♡

_____

_____

_____

_____

_____

_____

_____

_____

_____

⤫ Pick a goal (weight, clothes size, how you feel in your body, whatever you like). Write it down. ⤬

⤫ Keep your eyes on the blue skies of your own goal. ⤬
⤫ One small step after another. That's how you'll get there. ⤬
⤫ It truly does not matter how slowly you go as long as you don't stop. ⤬

⟫ Decide right now what you'll do when obstacles come ⟪

⤫ What will you do when obstacles come? Will you take care of yourself and keep striving for your goals or will you get derailed and give up? ⤬

⤫ Whatever your answer, now you know where you stand and what, if anything, you need to change. ⤬
⤫ Remember: mistakes are inevitable, defeat is optional. ⤬

⟫ Decide right now what you'll do when the temptation to quit comes ⟪

⤫ What will you do when the temptation to quit comes? Will you take care of yourself and keep striving for your goals or will you get derailed and give up? ⤬

⤫ Whatever your answer, now you know where you stand and what, if anything, you need to change. ⤬
⤫ Remember: mistakes are inevitable, defeat is optional. ⤬

·» Commit to being true to yourself «·

♡ Write a list of ways you have betrayed yourself. ♡

_____

_____

_____

_____

_____

_____

_____

♡ Are you willing to forgive yourself and begin again? Why or why not? ♡

_____

_____

_____

♡ Are you willing to commit to being true to yourself from this point forward? Why or why not? ♡

_____

_____

_____

  ♡ Remember: self-trust is paramount to your success. ♡

꙰ Will you commit to your own healing? Will you see your weight-loss journey through regardless of what comes up? Will you reach your goal(s) no matter how long it takes? Decide now. ꙰

_____

_____

_____

_____

꙰ Whatever your answers, now you know where you stand and what, if anything, you need to change. ꙰

꙰ If you've decided to commit to your own healing, to seeing your weight-loss journey through to the end, and/or to reaching your goals, write a note below giving yourself your word, committing to your own health and well-being and to not giving up on yourself. ꙰
꙰ Then sign your name and date. ꙰

_____

_____

_____

_____

_____

_____

_____

Name:_____**Date:**_____

꙰ Now honor and respect yourself by keeping your word to yourself. ꙰

·» Oh, some science «·

♡ What do you want/need to think about yourself or the task at hand to get to where you most want to be? ♡

_____

_____

_____

_____

_____

_____

_____

♡ What behaviors do you want/need to stop/start doing to get to where you most want to be? ♡

_____

_____

_____

_____

_____

_____

♡ Now mark your calendar for 66 days from today. ♡

♡ Then think one of those thoughts and do one of those behaviors every day. ♡

·» This is a practice and a process «·

♡ Are you willing to cherry pick from the information you've gotten, figure out what works for you, then do that? Why or why not? ♡

_____

_____

_____

♡ Are you willing to acknowledge that, no matter what you do, at some point you're going to make mistakes? Why or why not? ♡

_____

_____

_____

♡ Are you willing to give yourself unlimited tries to get it (whatever "it" is for you) right? If not, why not? ♡

_____

_____

_____

♡ Are you willing to forgive yourself when you make mistakes and simply start again? If not, why not? ♡

_____

_____

_____

♡ Say this aloud and believe it: Every mistake is simply a brand new chance to do it better the next time. ♡

❧ What worked for you during this chapter? What didn't? ☙

_____

_____

_____

_____

_____

_____

❧ Always, always, always find what works for you and do that. ☙
❧ You have permission to let go, right now and always, of anything that doesn't work for you. ☙

❧ Write a list of things you've learned from your mistakes. ☙

_____

_____

_____

_____

_____

_____

❧ Learn what you can, come at it again from a wiser perspective, then move on. ☙
❧ Remember: every mistake is simply a brand new chance to do it better the next time. ☙

Chapter Two!

·» Some beginning steps to take «·

·» Take the pressure off «·

♡ Write a list of outside reasons that make you feel pressured into shedding the weight and/or ceasing to abuse food? ♡

_____

_____

_____

_____

_____

_____

_____

♡ Are you willing, now and always, to make your own self and your own well-being the only reason you're shedding the weight and/or ceasing to abuse food? Why or why not? ♡

_____

_____

_____

♡ Remember: you're not doing it for them, you're doing it for you. ♡

♡ Are you willing to look at your life as an experiment or a game? Why or why not? ♡

_____

_____

_____

♡ Are you willing to take away the deadlines and the time tables as to when you'll be finished shedding the weight and/or ceasing to abuse food? Why or why not? ♡

_____

_____

_____

·» Put yourself at the top of your to-do list «·

♡ Write today's to-do list. Then write your name at the top of that list. ♡

_____

_____

_____

_____

_____

_____

_____

♡ Who are you living, doing, and making choices for on a regular basis, is it you? ♡

_____

_____

_____

♡ Why don't you think you're important enough to be number one on your own list of priorities? ♡

_____

_____

_____

_____

♡ Why do you believe that your wants and needs matter less than others? ♡

_____

_____

_____

♡ When will you look at your life as your own and take responsibility for your own happiness? ♡

_____

_____

_____

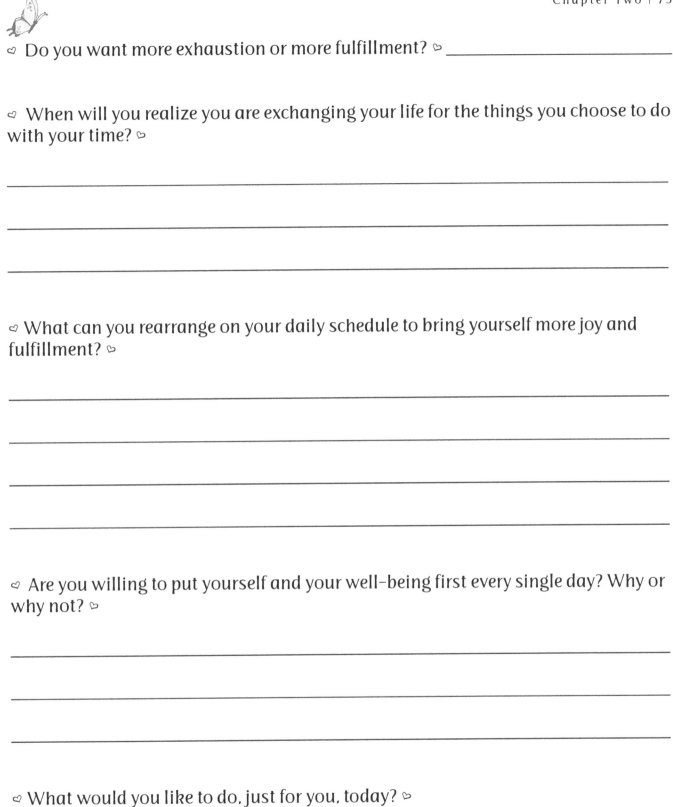

❦ Do you want more exhaustion or more fulfillment? ❧ _____

❦ When will you realize you are exchanging your life for the things you choose to do with your time? ❧

_____

_____

_____

❦ What can you rearrange on your daily schedule to bring yourself more joy and fulfillment? ❧

_____

_____

_____

_____

❦ Are you willing to put yourself and your well-being first every single day? Why or why not? ❧

_____

_____

_____

❦ What would you like to do, just for you, today? ❧

_____

_____

❦ Now go do it, guilt-free. Repeat daily. ❧

♡ Write this five times: No. ♡

1. _____

2. _____

3. _____

4. _____

5. _____

♡ Now remember:
no is a complete sentence. ♡

·» Take excellent care of yourself «·

♡ What do you most need to do today to improve your physical health? ♡

_____

_____

_____

♡ What do you most need to do today to improve your mental health? ♡

_____

_____

_____

♡ What do you most need to do today to improve your spiritual health? ♡

_____

_____

_____

♡ Now give yourself permission and go do those things to take care of your health today. ♡

·» Meet your own needs «·

♡ Determine where you fall on the needs hierarchy. ♡

_____

_____

♡ Which of your needs in that category are not being met? ♡

_____

_____

_____

_____

_____

♡ What do you need to have/be/do/say to meet those particular needs today? ♡

_____

_____

_____

_____

_____

_____

♡ Now take action and meet your own needs today. ♡

·» The crux of effective and permanent weight loss «·

·» Don't be possessive about food «·

♡ Have you been possessive about food? If so, how? Are you willing to stop? Why or why not? ♡

_____

_____

_____

_____

·» You are eating too much «·

♡ Do you believe you are eating too much? If not, are you willing to be open to the possibility that you are eating too much? Why or why not? ♡

_____

_____

_____

_____

♡ Do you acknowledge that the only one responsible for your weight is you? Why or why not? ♡

_____

_____

_____

_____

·⟩⟩ Eat when you're hungry ⟨⟨·

⊲ Are you willing to wait until you're hungry to eat? Why or why not? ⊳

_____

_____

_____

⊲ Describe what physiological hunger feels like for you. ⊳

_____

_____

_____

·⟩⟩ Eat calmly ⟨⟨·

⊲ Are you willing to do whatever you need to do for yourself so that you can eat calmly? Why or why not? ⊳

_____

_____

_____

⊲ Are you willing to pause, step away from the food, and ask yourself kindly: "What's the matter, [insert your name]? What do you need?" Why or why not? ⊳

_____

_____

❧ Are you willing to meet your own need(s) so you won't abuse food? Why or why not? ☙

_____

_____

_____

❧ Are you willing to feel whatever feelings come up in you without abusing food? Why or why not? ☙

_____

_____

_____

❧ Write a list of things you can (and would like) to do to interrupt the pattern in your brain where you abuse food as a solution to your emotions and/or problems. ☙

_____

_____

_____

_____

_____

_____

_____

_____

❧ Refer back to this list whenever you need to interrupt a pattern. ☙

·» Eat mindfully «·

♡ Are you willing to believe in the wisdom of your own body? Why or why not? ♡

_____

_____

_____

♡ Are you willing to eat mindfully and pay attention to your body for hunger/ fullness cues? Why or why not? ♡

_____

_____

_____

_____

♡ Write what fullness cues feel like in your body. ♡

_____

_____

_____

_____

♡ If you don't know yet, no worries, just pay attention. ♡

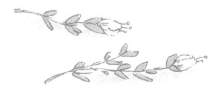

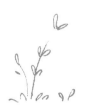

·» Eat whatever you want «·

❧ Does it feel like freedom or fear for you to not have a food plan and instead to eat whatever you want? Why? ☙

_____

_____

_____

_____

❧ Are you willing to listen to the wisdom of your body and eat whatever your body is craving? Why or why not? ☙

_____

_____

_____

❧ The next time you are hungry, answer these: What is your body craving right now? What exactly do you want to eat? ☙

_____

_____

❧ Now give yourself permission and go eat that. Stop when you are comfortably full. ☙

❧ Are you willing to heal yourself instead of harm yourself? Why or why not? ☙

_____

_____

_____

·» Eat exactly what you want «·

⟡ Write a list of foods that you know trigger binges for you. ⟡

_____

_____

_____

_____

_____

⟡ Now give yourself permission to not eat those foods for as long as you need to. ⟡

⟡ Do you believe there are good and bad foods? Why or why not? ⟡

_____

_____

_____

⟡ Are you willing to believe that there are no good and bad foods, that no foods are off-limits? Why or why not? ⟡

_____

_____

_____

⟡ Stop limiting yourself with that mindset. All you have to do is change your mind. ⟡

·» Eat only what tastes good «·

◁ Are you willing to eat only what tastes good? Why or why not? ▷

_____

_____

_____

◁ Are you willing to make eating a pleasing experience for yourself? Why or why not? ▷

_____

_____

_____

·» Drink when you're thirsty «·

◁ Are you willing to drink (not eat) when you're thirsty? Why or why not? ▷

_____

_____

_____

◁ Are you willing to only drink unsweetened drinks between meals? Why or why not? ▷

_____

_____

_____

·» Stop when you're comfortably full «·

⟡ Are you willing to stop eating when you are comfortably full? Why or why not? ⟡

_____

_____

_____

⟡ Do you believe that part of taking excellent care of yourself is deciding what you're going to put in or not put in your body? Why or why not? ⟡

_____

_____

_____

·» Get rid of the all-or-nothing thinking «·

⟡ Are you willing to cut yourself some slack when you make mistakes? Why or why not? ⟡

_____

_____

_____

⟡ Are you willing to do away with all-or-nothing thinking? Why or why not? ⟡

_____

_____

_____

⟡ You'll be doing yourself a kindness if you do. ⟡

❧ Write some ways that you can treat yourself with kindness. ☙

_____

_____

_____

_____

❧ Write words you really need to hear to reassure yourself. ☙

_____

_____

_____

_____

❧ Now say those words out loud (even better say them aloud looking at yourself in a mirror). ☙

❧ Are you willing to choose to take the pressure off and simply do better the next time? Why or why not? ☙

_____

_____

_____

❧ Are you willing to believe that weight loss and/or the cessation of abusing food really is as easy as you want to make it? Why or why not? ☙

_____

_____

_____

❧ It's just a matter of changing your mind. ☙

·» Some other suggestions to help you «·

⟡ What do you tell yourself when you justify eating when you're not hungry? ⟡

_____

_____

_____

⟡ Who are you justifying to? ⟡

_____

_____

⟡ Remember: you're not doing this for them, you're doing it for you. ⟡

·» Some things you're going to have to start doing «·

·» Relinquish your membership in the clean-plate club «·

⟡ Are you willing to stop finishing everything on your plate? If not, why not? ⟡

_____

_____

_____

⟡ Are you willing to: 1. serve yourself a lot less, 2. be okay with eating leftovers, or 3. start throwing away food when you're comfortably full? If not, why not? ⟡

_____

_____

_____

❧ Are you willing to believe, if you don't already, that you matter more and are worth more than food? Why or why not? ❧

_____

_____

_____

❧ Repeat this—I matter more and am worth more than food—until you believe it. ❧
❧ Remember: food is just fuel for your body so you can thrive. ❧

·» Move more (if you're not already getting some exercise) «·

❧ Are you willing to start small and build on an exercise routine? Why or why not? ❧

_____

_____

_____

❧ Are you willing to get out of the mindset of exercising solely to burn calories? If not, why not? ❧

_____

_____

_____

❧ Write this: I am exercising to be strong and feel better. ❧

_____

_____

❧ Say that out loud. Then say it aloud again. ❧
❧ Repeat as often as needed to get yourself moving more. ❧

♡ Write a list of exercises you enjoy. ♡

_____

_____

_____

_____

_____

_____

_____

♡ The right exercise for you is the one that you'll do, so pick one from that list and go do it today. ♡

♡ Do you believe patience is your friend? Why or why not? ♡

_____

_____

_____

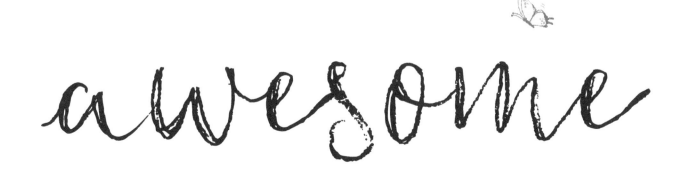

♡ Will you take full responsibility for how your life turns out? Why or why not? ♡

_____

_____

_____

♡ Write this: No one is coming to fix it. ♡

_____

_____

♡ Say that out loud. Then say it aloud again. ♡
♡ Repeat as often as needed to get yourself moving more. ♡

·» Discover what nonfood things nourish you «·

♡ Write any soul-crushing advice you've ever received? ♡

_____

_____

_____

_____

_____

_____

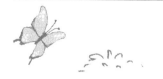

♡ Now ignore it. ♡

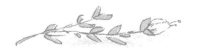

◌ Write a list of things and activities that you know nourish you. ◌

◌ Nourish means something that will build you up, help you grow, fulfill you,
and make you feel good about yourself and about being alive. ◌

_____

_____

_____

_____

_____

_____

_____

_____

◌ Write a list of any other things or activities that grab your attention. ◌

_____

_____

_____

_____

_____

❧ For each thing or activity that catches your attention, answer this: What do you (not anybody else) love about this? ❧

_____

_____

_____

_____

_____

_____

_____

❧ Trust yourself and pick one of those things or activities (the one you're most drawn to), give it a try, and see if it nourishes you. Write how it went. ❧

_____

_____

_____

_____

_____

_____

_____

❧ If it wasn't as nourishing as you thought, simply pick another thing/activity on your list and try again. ❧

·» Understand that food will never protect you from life «·

⊘ What, if anything, are you hoping that abusing food will fix in your life. ⊘

_____

_____

_____

_____

⊘ Write this five times: Food will not fix this. ⊘

1. _____

2. _____

3. _____

4. _____

5. _____

⊘ Now say it aloud five times: Food will not fix this. ⊘
⊘ Repeat until you take it to heart, believe it, and live your life by it. ⊘

·» Break your bad habits and make some good ones «·

⊘ What's your favorite part of your comfort zone? ⊘

_____

_____

_____

_____

☙ Are you afraid to leave your comfort zone? If so, why? ❧

_____

_____

_____

_____

_____

☙ Do you believe you're limited by your comfort zone? Why or why not? ❧

_____

_____

_____

☙ Are you open and willing to change and to make new habits? If not, why not? ❧

_____

_____

_____

☙ Do you believe your habits are under your control? Why or why not? ❧

_____

_____

_____

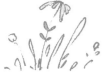
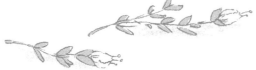

✐ Write a list of bad habits you know you have. ✐

_____

_____

_____

_____

_____

_____

✐ A bad habit is one that doesn't help you move forward. ✐

✐ Write a list of good habits you want to make. ✐

_____

_____

_____

_____

_____

_____

_____

_____

✐ Now repeat, repeat, repeat daily for 66 days ✐

·» Some notes on «·

·» Sabotaging yourself «·

◁ What are you afraid, anxious, concerned is going to happen when you lose the weight and/or stop abusing food? ▷

_____

_____

_____

_____

_____

_____

◁ What are you afraid, anxious, concerned you are going to have to do once you lose the weight and/or stop abusing food? ▷

_____

_____

_____

_____

_____

_____

_____

♡ Write a list of all the benefits you gain (or perceive you gain) by being overweight and/or abusing food. ♡

_____

_____

_____

_____

_____

_____

_____

♡ Write down the mistakes you made when you were so close to what you wanted. ♡

_____

_____

_____

_____

_____

_____

_____

꙰ Write down why you made those mistakes. ꙰

_____

_____

_____

_____

_____

_____

_____

_____

_____

_____

_____

꙰ Read all those answers and find the common thread running through them all. ꙰

꙰ Write that common thread down. ꙰

_____

_____

_____

_____

꙰ That common thread is likely your biggest fear. ꙰

⤳ **Eating disorders** ⤶

♡ Write this: I am so much more than a number on a scale. ♡

_____

_____

♡ Now say it aloud five times. ♡
♡ Repeat until you take it to heart, believe it, and live your life by it. ♡

♡ Write this: I have so much more to offer than the smallness of abusing food. ♡

_____

_____

♡ Now say it aloud five times. ♡
♡ Repeat until you take it to heart, believe it, and live your life by it. ♡

♡ Write this: I refuse to be trapped in a cycle. ♡

_____

_____

♡ Now say it aloud five times. ♡
♡ Repeat until you take it to heart, believe it, and live your life by it. ♡

♡ Write this: I believe that food is fuel so I can thrive. ♡

_____

_____

♡ Now say it aloud five times. ♡
♡ Repeat until you take it to heart, believe it, and live your life by it. ♡

❧ Write this: I am not doing this for anyone else; I am doing this for myself. ☙

_____

_____

❧ Now say it aloud five times. ☙
❧ Repeat until you take it to heart, believe it, and live your life by it. ☙

❧ Write this: I am doing this to save my own life. ☙

_____

_____

❧ Now say it aloud five times. ☙
❧ Repeat until you take it to heart, believe it, and live your life by it. ☙

❧ Do you believe you control food or does food control you? ☙

_____

_____

❧ Hint: if your life revolves around abusing food in some way then, I say kindly, food controls you. ☙

❧ Write a list of people whom you trust to help and support you. ☙

_____

_____

_____

_____

❧ Do yourself a kindness, reach out to one of them and ask for their help and support today. ☙

·» The scale «·

♡ Do you believe you're so much more than a number on a scale? If not, why not? ♡

_____

_____

_____

♡ Write this five times: I am so much more than a number on a scale. ♡

1. _____

2. _____

3. _____

4. _____

5. _____

♡ Now say it aloud five times. ♡
♡ Repeat until you take it to heart, believe it, and live your life by it. ♡

♡ Write some things you have to offer and/or that are awesome about you that have absolutely nothing to do with your weight. ♡

_____

_____

_____

_____

♡ Focus on and/or pursue those instead. ♡

⟩⟩ Encouragement and support groups ⟨⟨

❧ Do you believe you can lose weight and/or stop abusing food without a support system? Why or why not? ☙

_____

_____

_____

❧ Write what the ideal support system would look like to you. ☙

_____

_____

_____

❧ Seek that out. If you can't find it, then you must create it. ☙

❧ Write this: I am not in competition with anyone to reach my weight-loss and life goals. ☙

_____

_____

❧ Now say it aloud five times. ☙
❧ Repeat until you take it to heart, believe it, and live your life by it. ☙

brave

·» Recipes «·

ᴄ Write the names of some of your favorite recipes. ᴄ

_____

_____

_____

_____

_____

ᴄ Feel free to eat them when you're hungry and just stop eating when you're comfortably full. ᴄ

·» Oh, some science (part one) «·

ᴄ Are you willing to sit with your emotions and feel them for 90 seconds without abusing food and/or other substances/behaviors? Why or why not? ᴄ

_____

_____

_____

ᴄ It's a commitment to yourself to sit for those 90 seconds without abusing food. ᴄ

ᴄ Are you willing to sit with your emotions and feel them for 90 seconds and not dredge up your personal backstory? Why or why not? ᴄ

_____

_____

_____

ᴄ It's a commitment to yourself to not dredge up your history during those 90 seconds. ᴄ

♡ Are you willing to sit with your emotions and feel them for 90 seconds and learn about yourself? Why or why not? ♡

_____

_____

_____

♡ It's a commitment to yourself to learn about yourself during those 90 seconds. ♡

·» Oh, some science (part two) «·

♡ Write a list of (nonfood) things you can do to help calm yourself down. ♡

_____

_____

_____

_____

_____

_____

_____

_____

_____

♡ Refer back to this list whenever you need to ease your mind. ♡

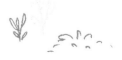

·» This is a practice and a process «·

✎ What worked for you during this chapter? What didn't? ✎

_____

_____

_____

_____

_____

_____

✎ Always, always, always find what works for you and do that. ✎
✎ You have permission to let go, right now, of anything that doesn't work for you. ✎

✎ Write a list of things you've learned from your mistakes. ✎

_____

_____

_____

_____

_____

✎ Learn what you can, come at it again from a wiser perspective, then move on. ✎
✎ Remember: every mistake is simply a brand new chance to do it better the next time. ✎

Chapter Three!

·» Something you need to know «·

♡ Be honest: Would you put your life in the hands of someone you didn't trust? Why or why not? ♡

_____

_____

_____

♡ Do you believe your life is already in your hands? Why or why not? ♡

_____

_____

_____

♡ Your life is already in your hands. It's up to you how you want to live it. ♡

♡ Write an instance when you listened to your intuition and did what it said regardless of the advice of others. What was the outcome? Was the outcome what you'd hoped it would be? ♡

_____

_____

_____

❥ Write an instance when you refused to listen to your intuition and listened to someone else's advice instead? What was the outcome? Was the outcome what you'd hoped it would be? ❧

_____

_____

_____

_____

_____

·» Things you need to do to build your self-trust «·

·» Practice self-compassion «·

❥ Write your life story by jotting down experiences: a memory here, a memory there (especially any memories that have a strong emotional connection/reaction). ❧

_____

_____

_____

_____

_____

_____

_____

_____

◁ Your life story continued. ▷

_____

_____

_____

_____

_____

_____

_____

_____

_____

_____

_____

_____

_____

_____

_____

◁ This will separate your story from yourself so you can look at your life objectively. ▷

ᴄ Now read the life story you just wrote. ᴆ
ᴄ See all the places where you were so much stronger than whatever it was that tried to defeat you. ᴆ

ᴄ Now write down what each of those experiences taught you. ᴆ

_____

_____

_____

_____

_____

_____

_____

_____

_____

_____

_____

_____

_____

_____

ᴄ Realize that each of those experiences served a purpose in your life as lessons about yourself or others. ᴆ

·» Listen to your own intuition «·

∽ Do you believe your intuition will never tear you down or berate you or harm you? Do you believe your intuition will always encourage you, strengthen you, and help you grow? Why or why not? ∾

_____

_____

_____

∽ Do you believe in the power of your own intuition? Why or why not? ∾

_____

_____

_____

∽ Do you believe you empower yourself by listening and acting upon your own intuition? Why or why not? ∾

_____

_____

_____

∽ Are you willing to trust your intuition implicitly? Why or why not? ∾

_____

_____

_____

∽ Do what your intuition guides you to do every single time, and you'll come to trust yourself implicitly. ∾
∽ Going against your intuition is an act of self-betrayal. ∾

Think of some choices you're facing that you're conflicted as to what to do. Now answer this: What feels (deep down, where it's quiet and still) like the right thing to do?

_____

_____

_____

_____

_____

_____

_____

_____

_____

_____

_____

_____

_____

_____

Your intuition will guide you to what's good for you and what you need to do to fulfill yourself.

What matters most is that you're moving in the direction your intuition tells you to go.

❧ Write a list of instances when you didn't listen to your intuition for whatever reason. How did each turn out? Was it how you'd hoped or expected? ☙

_____

_____

_____

_____

_____

_____

_____

_____

❧ Write a list of instances when you trusted yourself and listened to your intuition and did what it said. How did each turn out? Was it how you'd hoped or expected? ☙

_____

_____

_____

_____

_____

_____

_____

_____

·» The excess weight/food abuse is just a barometer «·

♡ Are you willing to be open to the idea that all the excess weight and/or food abuse is simply showing you that you need to strengthen and fortify your self-trust? Why or why not? ♡

_____

_____

_____

♡ What's happening in your life (past, present, and/or future) that you don't trust yourself to handle either emotionally or physically? ♡

_____

_____

_____

_____

_____

♡ In what areas of your life do you not much trust yourself? ♡

_____

_____

_____

_____

·» Change what you believe «·

۰ Do you believe self-trust starts with what you believe about yourself? Why or why not? ۰

_____

_____

_____

۰ Do you agree that you will live out whatever it is you believe about yourself? Why or why not? ۰

_____

_____

_____

۰ Write a list of thoughts/beliefs you have about yourself. ۰

_____

_____

_____

_____

_____

_____

_____

۰ Now beside each one, write an answer to these: Is that true or false? Does it strengthen me or weaken me? Do I even want that thought/belief in my head? ۰

⚮ Reading over that list, do you think mostly good things or mostly bad things about yourself? ⚮

_____

⚮ Pay attention to how your body feels when you read that list. Do you feel energized or drained? ⚮

⚮ You can accept or reject any thought/belief that you want; that choice is always up to you. ⚮

⚮ Write a list of thoughts/beliefs that will strengthen you and/or better serve you. ⚮

_____

_____

_____

_____

_____

_____

_____

_____

_____

_____

⚮ Repeat (repeat, repeat) thoughts that strengthen you until they become the beliefs that guide you. ⚮

·» **Always keep your word to yourself** «·

⌁ Do you think it's important to keep your word to yourself? Why or why not? ⌃

_____

_____

_____

⌁ Are you willing to keep your word to yourself every single time? Why or why not? ⌃

_____

_____

_____

⌁ You committed to yourself back in Chapter One (page 66). Now write a note recommitting to yourself and giving yourself your word that you're on this journey for the long haul and you will see it all the way through to the end. ⌃
⌁ Include things like: you're going to stay at it until you find what works for you, you will have your own back always, you won't give up on yourself no matter what. Then sign your name and date. ⌃

_____

_____

_____

_____

_____

Name:_____**Date:**_____

⌁ Honor yourself and keep your word to yourself. ⌃

·» Manage your disappointment (and other feelings) without food «·

♡ Do you believe food will fix your disappointment? Why or why not? ♡

_____

_____

_____

♡ Write a list of things that have disappointed you, including yourself. ♡

_____

_____

_____

_____

_____

♡ Sit with all those disappointments and really feel them for 90 seconds
without abusing food or anything else to numb yourself. Then let those feelings go. ♡

♡ Now write what actions you can take (even if they're tiny steps) to get you moving
in the direction you want to go. ♡

_____

_____

_____

_____

·» Choose you «·

⊙ Are you willing to choose to make yourself happy and fulfilled regardless of what anyone else does or doesn't do for you? Why or why not? ☙

_____

_____

_____

⊙ Are you willing to choose yourself and what matters to you even if (especially if) no one else chooses you? Why or why not? ☙

_____

_____

_____

⊙ Every time you choose yourself, you will trust yourself a little bit more. ☙

·» Change how you value yourself «·

⊙ Do you value yourself? Why or why not? ☙

_____

_____

_____

♡ Food is fuel. What other things are you looking for food to do for you? ♡

♡ For example: emotional support, validation, feelings of importance, etc. ♡

_____

_____

_____

_____

♡ What measurement, if any, are you using to place worth and value on yourself? ♡

♡ For example: hours you spend at the gym, what the scale said today, how much money you make, etc. ♡

_____

_____

_____

_____

♡ Write this: My worth and value are innate. I have worth and value because I am alive. ♡

_____

_____

_____

♡ Now say it aloud. Take it to heart and believe it. ♡

♡ Write this: What I say and do matters because I matter. ♡

_____

_____

♡ Now say it aloud. Take it to heart and believe it. ♡

✑ Write a few of your gifts/talents/passions/interests. ✑

_____

_____

_____

✑ Prioritize and cultivate those. ✑

·» Like yourself «·

✑ Do you like yourself? Why or why not? ✑

_____

_____

_____

✑ In what ways have you been mean to yourself? ✑

_____

_____

_____

✑ Write a list of things that are awesome and likeable about you. ✑

_____

_____

_____

✑ Now go do something nice for yourself, something you would really like to have/do. ✑

·» Be your own best friend «·

৶ Are you willing to be for yourself the kind of best friend you've always wanted to have? Why or why not? ৬

_____

_____

_____

৶ Describe your ideal best friend. What traits does that person have? ৬

৶ For example: loyalty, honesty, loves you no matter what, etc. ৬

_____

_____

_____

_____

_____

৶ Are you willing to have those same traits with yourself? If not, why not and what do you need to do to change your mind? ৬

_____

_____

_____

_____

৶ Now go be the best friend to yourself that you could ever have. ৬

·» Empower yourself by being the authority in your own life «·

⊲ Do you BELIEVE you are the authority in your own life? Why or why not? ⊳

_____

_____

_____

⊲ Do you ACT like you are the authority in your own life? Why or why not? ⊳
⊲ For example: do you sneak food, not wait until you're hungry to eat, not stop when you're full, justify why you're abusing food, refuse to find an exercise you enjoy, etc. ⊳

_____

_____

_____

⊲ Do you agree it's your lack of self-trust that makes you feel powerless? Why or why not? ⊳

_____

_____

_____

⊲ Have you given up power over your own life? If yes, in what areas? ⊳

_____

_____

_____

Do you believe abusing food will give you control over your own life? Why or why not?

_____

_____

_____

Do you believe you have given food your power? Why or why not?

_____

_____

_____

Do you believe you have the power to fix your own life? Why or why not?

_____

_____

_____

Do you believe all the choices are still yours and no one else's? Why or why not?

_____

_____

_____

⊘ What choices do you know you need to make and/or actions you know you need to take but are scared to do so? ⊳

_____

_____

_____

_____

⊘ No one is coming. ⊳
⊘ The only way to get your power back is to take it. So take it back. ⊳

·» Realize that you can never get enough of what you don't need «·

⊘ When you want to abuse food: Pause. Breathe. Listen for your intuition. Then answer: ⊳
⊘ What's the matter? ⊳
⊘ Start at right now and move backward to that moment of the stimulus (what triggered your desire to abuse food). What were you feeling at the point of the stimulus and why? ⊳

_____

_____

_____

_____

_____

_____

⊘ Let yourself fully feel the emotion(s) that are coming up in you. ⊳

৶ When you want to abuse food: Pause. Breathe. Listen for your intuition. Then answer: ৯

৶ What do you need? (really need—not food-related—instead of abusing food) ৯

৶ Trust yourself to know. ৯

_____

_____

_____

_____

_____

_____

_____

_____

৶ Now take action to do whatever it takes to meet that need(s) for yourself. ৯
৶ And watch your self-trust grow. ৯

·» Quit procrastinating «·

৶ Write a list of activities/people/things that you are putting off? ৯

_____

_____

_____

_____

_____

❧ For each item on your list, answer this: What am I afraid of? ❧

_____

_____

_____

_____

_____

❧ Read through the answers you just wrote. Find the thread that connects them. Write it here. ❧

_____

_____

❧ That thread is likely your biggest fear. ❧

❧ What's the tiniest step you can take to get you moving through that biggest fear? ❧

_____

_____

❧ Take that step today. ❧

❧ What's the next tiniest step you can take after that? ❧

_____

_____

❧ Take that step today. ❧
❧ The only thing you have to do when fear happens is to take a deep breath then take the next step. ❧

·» Determine whose voice is in your head «·

⊘ Pause. Breathe. Listen for your intuition. Then answer: ⊘
⊘ What negative words/phrases are echoing around in your head? ⊘

_____

_____

_____

_____

_____

_____

⊘ For each, answer this: Whose voice(s) do those words actually belong to? ⊘
⊘ Now circle any words/phrases coming from a voice that isn't wholly yours. ⊘

⊘ How is it serving you to allow these other people's voices in your head? What do you hope to gain? ⊘

_____

_____

_____

_____

⊘ Choose to reject any voice that isn't serving you. ⊘
⊘ It is your head after all. You're the one that gets to edit what it's thinking. ⊘

♡ Listen for your own voice: the quieter one that is kinder to you, the soft-spoken one that believes in you, the one that does not (and never will) berate you or tear you down. ♡

♡ Write down what it says about you, your chances, your place in the world, etc. ♡

_____

_____

_____

_____

_____

_____

_____

_____

_____

_____

_____

_____

_____

_____

_____

♡ Repeat, repeat, repeat what that voice (your own voice) has to say about you. ♡
♡ You are only what you say and think and believe about yourself. ♡

·» Speak strength to yourself «·

ᴄ You will live out whatever it is you're repeating to yourself. ᴄ

ᴄ Pick three words that give you strength and feel expansive when you use them to describe yourself. ᴄ

I am _____

I am _____

I am _____

ᴄ Look yourself in the eyes in a mirror every morning for at least 66 days and say those words to yourself. ᴄ

ᴄ Repeat (repeat, repeat) those words throughout the day. ᴄ

·» Relax into it «·

ᴄ Do you believe you can do anything if you'll just relax into it? Why or why not? ᴄ

_____

_____

_____

·» Settle in to the in-between «·

ᴄ Have you been able to let that in-between space motivate you instead of scare you? Why or why not? (See your answer on page 45) ᴄ

_____

_____

_____

·» Refuse to give up on yourself «·

♡ Do you believe you can conquer anything if you'll just refuse to quit? Why or why not? ♡

_____

_____

_____

♡ Your self-trust will become a rock-solid foundation when you steadfastly refuse to give up on yourself. ♡

·» A special note for survivors of abuse «·

·» Fat tissue and abusing food are poor substitutes «·

♡ If you are overweight, do you believe the fat tissue will protect you? Why or why not? ♡

_____

_____

_____

♡ If you believe that, what will you do when the fat tissue does not protect you? ♡

_____

_____

_____

ↅ Do you believe abusing food gives you power/control? Why or why not? ↄ

_____

_____

_____

ↅ If you believe that, what will you do when abusing food does not give you power/control? ↄ

_____

_____

_____

ↅ Write this: I have a right to defend myself and my body against anyone or anything that would harm me. ↄ

_____

_____

_____

ↅ Say that to yourself out loud. ↄ
ↅ Take that into your heart and believe it because it's absolutely true. ↄ

ↅ Are you willing to take a self-defense class? Why or why not? ↄ

_____

_____

_____

 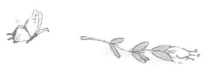 ↅ You are worth defending. ↄ

·❀ Some things you're likely trying to numb with food ❀·

·❀ Shame ❀·

✧ Shame says: I am bad, I shouldn't be who I am. ✧

✧ Are you caught in secret shame? If so, what do you feel shame about? ✧

✧ Remember: you don't have to show this to anyone until you're ready. So be honest. ✧

_____

_____

_____

_____

_____

_____

_____

_____

_____

_____

_____

_____

_____

_____

_____

_____

In case you need more space to write what you feel shame about. Get it all out. This is a safe place.

_____

_____

_____

_____

_____

_____

_____

_____

_____

_____

_____

_____

_____

_____

_____

_____

_____

❧ Write a list of people whom you trust. ❧

_____

_____

_____

_____

❧ Pick the one you trust the most. Tell them about your secret shame. ❧

❧ Write this: That's something that happened to me; it's not who I choose to be. ❧

_____

_____

❧ Write this: I lived through it because I am strong. ❧

_____

_____

❧ Write this: They tried to break me, but I'm not broken. ❧

_____

_____

❧ Write this: Food will not fix it. ❧

_____

_____

◌ Write this: I am proud of myself. I am strong. I have nothing to be ashamed of. ◌

_____

_____

◌ Now befriend yourself and say out loud all of those phrases you just wrote. ◌
◌ Be proud and protective of yourself always. ◌

◌ Do you believe shame is just a prison of your own making? Why or why not? ◌

_____

_____

_____

◌ Write a list of any other ideas, dreams, passions, and goals that move you toward the life you most want. (Add here to the list from page 118) ◌

_____

_____

_____

_____

_____

_____

_____

 ◌ Let those things fill the space that shame took up in your life. ◌

⸬» **Vulnerability (otherwise known as being your real self)** «⸬

৩ Do you let others see the real you? Why or why not? ৩

_____

_____

_____

৩ What are you afraid is going to happen if you show your real self to the world? ৩

_____

_____

_____

৩ Are you willing to free yourself from that fear so you can be yourself? Why or why not? ৩

_____

_____

_____

৩ You free yourself by showing up in the world as your real self. ৩

৩ Do you agree the biggest part of self-trust is being your authentic self all the time? Why or why not? ৩

_____

_____

_____

·» Rejection «·

♡ Take a deep breath. ♡
♡ Write a list of instances when you were rejected. ♡

_____

_____

_____

_____

_____

_____

♡ How did you handle each one? ♡

_____

_____

_____

_____

_____

_____

♡ Write who you are at your core: what you believe, what matters to you, what you stand for. ♡

_____

_____

_____

_____

_____

_____

_____

♡ Now don't back down or waver or hide those things from the world. ♡
♡ People who value the same things as you will gravitate toward you. ♡

♡ Have you ever rejected yourself? If so, how? ♡

_____

_____

_____

_____

♡ Are you willing to accept all of you as you are right now? Why or why not? ♡

_____

_____

_____

♡ If you don't, you'll just keep causing yourself pain. ♡

♡ Are you willing to look at rejection as an event and not as something personal about you? Why or why not? ♡

_____

_____

_____

♡ Are you willing to consider the possibility that rejections are just a way for you to stop heading down a path you aren't supposed to be on at that moment? Why or why not? ♡

_____

_____

_____

·» Lack of control «·

♡ Write a list of people, places, things, situations, outcomes, etc. that you're trying to control. ♡

_____

_____

_____

_____

_____

_____

♡ Remember: there are no guarantees of either security or comfort in nature. ♡

⊘ Are you willing to be okay with not knowing everything ahead of time? Why or why not? ⊖

_____

_____

_____

⊘ Are you willing to embrace change? Why or why not? ⊖

_____

_____

_____

⊘ Are you willing to believe, deep down, that you're strong enough to deal with whatever comes your way? Why or why not? ⊖

_____

_____

_____

⊘ Are you willing to consider the possibility that everything that's happening in your life is somehow working out for your good? Why or why not? ⊖

_____

_____

_____

❧ Write an instance when something bad happened that turned out to be something for your good. ❧

_____

_____

_____

_____

❧ Are you willing to fix what you can then start looking for the lesson in what you can't? Why or why not? ❧

_____

_____

_____

·» Fear «·

❧ Write something you really (maybe even desperately) want to have/be/do/say but the thought of having/being/doing/saying it also scares you tremendously. ❧

_____

_____

_____

_____

❧ Now sit with all those feelings of fear and really feel the fear for 90 seconds. ❧
❧ Take note: you're still alive; nothing bad happened to you by feeling the fear. ❧

♡ Write an instance when you didn't let real fear stop you. What was the outcome? ♡

_____

_____

_____

_____

♡ Write an instance when head fear stopped you. What was the outcome? ♡

_____

_____

_____

_____

♡ Do you agree that beyond head fear is where you will find freedom? Why or why not? ♡

_____

_____

_____

strong

♥ Start with your answer for something you really want to have/be/do/say (on page 139). ♥

♥ What steps do you need to take to move right through that fear? ♥

_____

_____

_____

_____

_____

_____

_____

_____

_____

_____

_____

_____

_____

_____

♥ Take a deep breath in through your nose, hold it three seconds, let it out slowly through your mouth. ♥

♥ Now take the first step (tiny, if need be) through that fear. ♥

·» Oh, some science (part one) «·

♡ Listen for your intuition. ♡
♡ What beliefs do you have that are holding you back?
♡ About yourself, about life in general, about your place in the world, about others, about your own gifts and talents, about your chances, and/or about anything else you'd like to address. ♡

_____

_____

_____

_____

_____

_____

_____

_____

_____

_____

_____

_____

_____

_____

_____

♡ Listen for your intuition. ♡
♡ What would you rather believe instead that'll help you? ♡

_____

_____

_____

_____

_____

_____

_____

_____

_____

_____

_____

_____

_____

_____

_____

♡ Now repeat those new thoughts over and over again until they become the beliefs that guide you. ♡

·» Oh, some science (part two) «·

♡ Are you willing to question not only the actual truth of but also your feelings about the thoughts, beliefs, and story/stories circling in your mind? Why or why not? ♡

_____

_____

_____

♡ Remember: you will live out what you believe to be true. ♡

♡ Write a thought/belief/story that's holding you back that you also feel is true. ♡

_____

_____

_____

_____

_____

_____

_____

◌ Now question that thought/belief/story that's holding you back. Is it actually true? Do you have evidence/proof that it is true? ◌

_____

_____

_____

_____

◌ If you do have evidence, how can you change how you feel about that evidence/proof so that you can overcome what's holding you back? ◌

_____

_____

_____

_____

◌ If you don't have evidence, why do you feel it is true? How can you change how you feel about that thought/belief/story so you can free yourself from it? ◌

_____

_____

_____

_____

_____

_____

·» This is a practice and a process «·

⊲ What worked for you during this chapter? What didn't? ⊳

_____

_____

_____

_____

_____

_____

⊲ Always, always, always find what works for you and do that. ⊳
⊲ You have permission to let go, right now, of anything that doesn't work for you. ⊳

⊲ Write a list of things you've learned from your mistakes. ⊳

_____

_____

_____

_____

_____

_____

⊲ Learn what you can, come at it again from a wiser perspective, then move on. ⊳
⊲ Remember: every mistake is simply a brand new chance to do it better the next time. ⊳

·» Notes or doodles «·

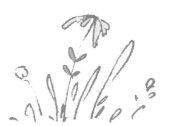

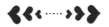

Chapter Four!

·» Change is your friend «·

♡ Are you open to believing (if you don't already) that whatever happened in the past, is currently happening now, and will happen in the future is somehow working out for your good? Why or why not? ♡

_____

_____

_____

♡ Write another instance when something you thought was really bad for you actually turned out to be something really good for you. ♡

_____

_____

_____

♡ Do you believe that you will grow and be stronger because of whatever happens to you? Why or why not? ♡

_____

_____

ᴗ Write an instance when you grew and became stronger because of something that happened to you. ᴗ

_____

_____

_____

_____

ᴗ Do you believe deep down in your core that you can take care of yourself no matter what happens? Why or why not? ᴗ

_____

_____

_____

ᴗ Write an instance when you took care of yourself when you weren't sure if you could. ᴗ

_____

_____

_____

ᴗ Are you willing to be the one to change, release your vice grip on all those things that no longer serve you, and let them go? Why or why not? ᴗ

_____

_____

_____

·» Things you're going to have to let go of «·

·» Using food as a crutch «·

♡ Take a deep breath. ♡
♡ Write a list of instances when you used food as a crutch. ♡

_____

_____

_____

_____

_____

♡ Why did you abuse food in each of those instances? ♡

_____

_____

_____

_____

_____

♡ Are you willing to let go of food as a crutch? Why or why not? ♡

_____

_____

_____

❧ Do you believe you are brave, tenacious, strong, intelligent, and you have everything it takes to achieve everything you want ? Why or why not? ❧

_____

_____

_____

❧ Write strength to yourself in the form of words you most need to hear right now. ❧

_____

_____

_____

❧ Now say them out loud (better yet while looking at yourself in a mirror) and believe them. ❧

❧ Write this: Food will not fix it. ❧

_____

❧ Are you willing to pause when you want to abuse food and ask yourself what is the matter? Are you willing to feel whatever emotions come up in you? Why or why not? ❧

_____

_____

_____

❧ Let yourself feel, for 90 seconds, whatever emotion(s) are causing you to want to abuse food. ❧

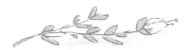 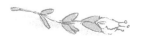 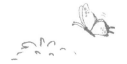

↺ Are you willing to pause when you want to abuse food and ask yourself what you need? Are you willing to do whatever is necessary to meet those needs? Why or why not? ↻

_____

_____

_____

↺ How is using food as a crutch serving you? Is it helping you or harming you? ↻

_____

_____

_____

↺ What do you believe food is doing for you? ↻

_____

_____

_____

↺ Now go do that thing(s) for yourself. ↻

↺ What do you need instead of food to fix the situation you're in? ↻

_____

_____

_____

↺ Now take action to meet your own need. ↻

❧ Are you willing to separate your emotions from food? Why or why not? ❧

_____

_____

_____

❧ Remember: food is just fuel for your body. ❧

❧ Write one action you can take to move yourself in the direction you most want your life to go. ❧

_____

_____

❧ Now take that action today. ❧

·» Having a scarcity mentality «·

❧ How is having a scarcity mentality serving you? Is it helping you or harming you? ❧

_____

_____

_____

❧ Take a deep breath. ❧
❧ Do you believe there is more than enough for you? Why or why not? ❧

_____

_____

_____

৶ Are you willing to believe in abundance? Why or why not? ৸

_____

_____

_____

৶ Write this: Life is on my side. ৸

_____

৶ Write this: There's more than enough for me. ৸

_____

_____

৶ Write this: I get everything I need. ৸

_____

৶ Now take those three phrases to heart. ৸
৶ Repeat them until they become the story that you live out in your life. ৸

৶ Write five things you are grateful for in your life today. ৸

1. _____

2. _____

3. _____

4. _____

5. _____

৶ Now add one item to that list every day (pages to do so start on page 392). ৸

·» Your failures «·

◃ How is holding on to your failures serving you? Is it helping you or harming you? ▹

_____

_____

_____

◃ Are you willing stop believing in failure? Why or why not? ▹

_____

_____

_____

◃ Take a deep breath. ▹
◃ Write a list of instances where you failed at something you tried to do. ▹

_____

_____

_____

_____

_____

_____

◃ Now take another deep breath. ▹

୭ Write what you learned from each one of those failures. ଡ

_____

_____

_____

_____

_____

_____

_____

୭ Each one of those lessons is a gift to you. ଡ

୭ Are you willing to reframe events so that you've got only two choices from now on: either you're going to succeed or you're going to learn? Why or why not? ଡ

_____

_____

_____

୭ Remember: you get unlimited tries. ଡ

୭ Write this: I believe there's only success or learning. ଡ

_____

_____

୭ Take that to heart, let yourself grow, and be extra kind to yourself as you move forward. ଡ

·» The past and what happened to you and who you used to be «·

♡ How is holding on to your past and what happened to you and who you used to be serving you? Is it helping you or harming you? ♡

_____

_____

_____

♡ Do you believe you hold on to your history at the expense of your present and your future? Why or why not? ♡

_____

_____

_____

♡ Take a deep breath. ♡
♡ Write a list of instances where you wish you could change something you did or didn't do. ♡

_____

_____

_____

_____

_____

_____

❧ For each instance you wish you could change, write a new story. Reframe each event in a different light. ❧

_____

_____

_____

_____

_____

_____

_____

_____

_____

_____

_____

_____

_____

_____

_____

_____

❧ Remember: you live out the story that you believe about yourself. ❧
❧ You can edit that story at any time. ❧

·» Regret and lost time «·

♡ How is holding on to regret and lost time serving you? Is it helping you or harming you? ♡

_____

_____

_____

♡ Take a deep breath. ♡
♡ Write a list of instances where you regret something you did or didn't do. ♡

_____

_____

_____

_____

_____

_____

_____

_____

_____

♡ Know this: all the regret in the world won't change a single thing. ♡

♡ For each instance you regret, write what you can learn from it. ♡

_____

_____

_____

_____

_____

_____

_____

_____

_____

_____

_____

_____

_____

_____

_____

_____

_____

꒰ Do you believe your history doesn't define you unless you let it? Why or why not? ꒱

_____

_____

_____

꒰ You wouldn't be the strong, determined, tenacious person you are today if not for your history. ꒱

꒰ Are you willing to believe that there is no lost time? Why or why not? ꒱

_____

_____

_____

·» Who you think you should be by now and/or what you think your life should look like by now «·

꒰ How is holding on to who you think you should be by now and/or what you think your life should look like by now serving you? Is it helping you or harming you? ꒱

_____

_____

_____

amazing

⊲ Take a deep breath. ⊳
⊲ Write a list/story of where you thought you would be right now in your life. ⊳

_____

_____

_____

_____

_____

_____

⊲ Are you willing to accept that your life is not yet the way you want to it be? Why or why not? ⊳

_____

_____

_____

⊲ Write this: I accept who I am right now. ⊳

_____

_____

⊲ Write this: I accept where I am right now. ⊳

_____

_____

⊲ Now say those two phrases out loud. ⊳
⊲ The insatiable want to abuse food will ease once you come to accept your life. ⊳

·» Someone else's idea of success «·

♥ How is holding on to someone else's idea of success serving you? Is it helping you or harming you? ♥

_____

_____

_____

♥ Are you willing to define success for yourself instead of listening to others? Why or why not? ♥

_____

_____

_____

♥ Take a deep breath. ♥
♥ Listen to your intuition and write a list of what deeply matters to you and is most important to you. ♥

_____

_____

_____

_____

_____

_____

◁ Using what deeply matters and is important to you, write your definition of success and what a successful life looks like to you. ▷

_____

_____

_____

_____

_____

_____

_____

_____

_____

_____

◁ Let your definition of success be your focus. ▷
◁ Now get busy working on achieving your own ideal of success. ▷

⇢ Comparison ⇠

◁ How is comparison serving you? Is it helping you or harming you? ▷

_____

_____

_____

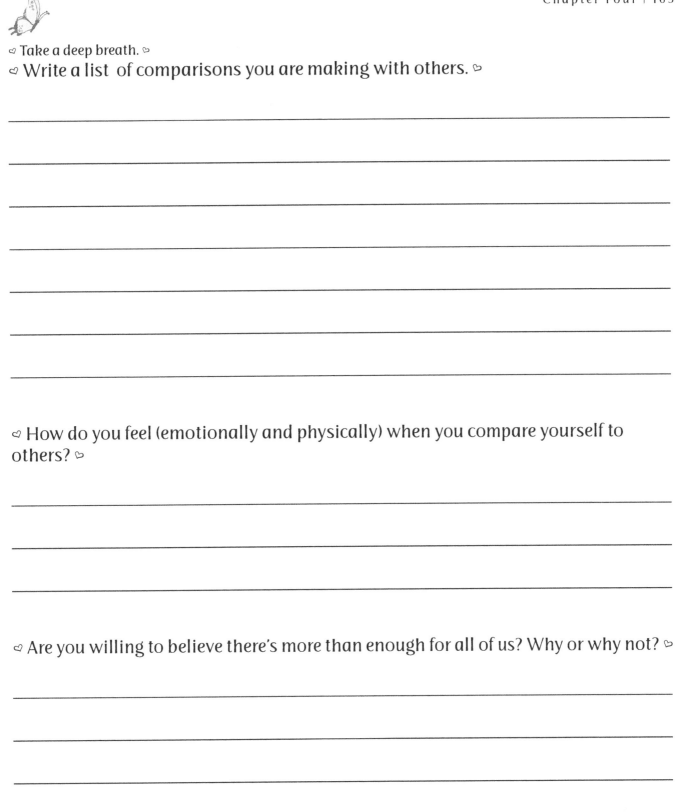

♡ Take a deep breath. ♡
♡ Write a list of comparisons you are making with others. ♡

_____

_____

_____

_____

_____

_____

♡ How do you feel (emotionally and physically) when you compare yourself to others? ♡

_____

_____

_____

♡ Are you willing to believe there's more than enough for all of us? Why or why not? ♡

_____

_____

_____

Do you believe you're capable of achieving what you most want from your life and of becoming the person you most want to be? Why or why not?

_____

_____

_____

You will always live out what you believe.
If you don't like what you believe, all you have to do is change your mind.

Write this: I believe in abundance. I believe there is more than enough for me. I believe in more life for everybody.

_____

_____

_____

_____

_____

Say that out loud. Believe it.
Repeat until it becomes the story that you live out in your life.
Now get busy creating the life you want.

·» Pretending to yourself «·

How is pretending to yourself serving you? Is it helping you or harming you?

_____

_____

_____

❧ Are you willing to be completely honest with yourself? Why or why not? ❧

_____

_____

_____

❧ Take a deep breath. ❧

❧ Write down the way your life is right now. Career. Finances. Relationships. Family. Education. Goals (reached and unreached). Dreams (fulfilled and unfulfilled). The status of your weight loss. Add anything else important to you. ❧

_____

_____

_____

_____

_____

_____

_____

_____

_____

_____

❧ This is who you are. This is where you are. Period. And that's okay. ❧
❧ Now you can truly just start where you are. ❧

♡ Write what choices/changes you need to make and what actions you need to take to make your reality a place where you actually want to live. ♡

_____

_____

_____

_____

_____

_____

_____

_____

_____

_____

_____

_____

_____

_____

_____

_____

♡ Now honor yourself and make/take them. ♡

·» **Lying to others** «·

◌ How is lying to others serving you? Is it helping you or harming you? ◌

_____

_____

_____

◌ Take a deep breath. ◌
◌ Now write the honest-to-goodness truth about what you do, who you are, what you want, and what you really love. ◌

_____

_____

_____

_____

_____

_____

_____

_____

_____

_____

◌ Know this: your preferences, whatever they may be, are okay. ◌

◌ Take a deep breath. ◌
◌ More space to write the honest-to-goodness truth. ◌

⊘ Are you willing to speak that truth aloud to yourself and to others? Why or why not? ⊵

_____

_____

_____

⊘ Are you willing to act that out in your life by pursuing what deeply matters to you? Why or why not? ⊵

_____

_____

_____

⊘ Write this: I am saving my own life by telling the truth about who I am. ⊵

_____

_____

_____

⊘ Say that out loud. Believe it. Repeat it until it becomes the story that you live out in your life. ⊵
⊘ Stand strong, hold your ground, and tell the truth. ⊵

·» Self-doubt «·

⊘ How is self-doubt serving you? Is it helping you or harming you? ⊵

_____

_____

_____

♡ Take a deep breath. ♡
♡ Write a list of any failures that may be fueling the self-doubt you feel. ♡

_____

_____

_____

_____

♡ Take a deep breath. ♡
♡ Write a list of any criticisms that may be fueling the self-doubt you feel. ♡

_____

_____

_____

_____

♡ Take a deep breath. ♡
♡ Write a list of any comparisons that may be fueling the self-doubt you feel. ♡

_____

_____

_____

_____

❧ Are you willing to believe that self-doubt is a self-worth issue? Why or why not? ☙

_____

_____

_____

❧ Write what you want to believe about yourself. ☙

_____

_____

_____

_____

_____

_____

_____

_____

_____

❧ Write a list of your weaknesses that you may be playing to. ☙

_____

_____

_____

_____

☙ Write a list of your strengths that you can play to instead. ❧

_____

_____

_____

_____

_____

❧ Focus on improving, growing, and mastering your strengths. ❧

☙ Are you willing to hire/barter with others where your skills are weak? Why or why not? ❧

_____

_____

_____

☙ Are you willing to persevere until you finish and prove to yourself just how capable, strong, intelligent, committed, and determined you are? Why or why not? ❧

_____

_____

_____

·» Self-abuse «·

⌁ Take a deep breath. ⌁

⌁ How is self-abuse serving you? Is it helping you or harming you? ⌁

_____

_____

_____

⌁ Do you believe self-abuse is self-betrayal? Why or why not? ⌁

_____

_____

_____

⌁ Are you willing to choose to befriend yourself, have self-compassion, and believe in your own worth and value all the time? Why or why not? ⌁

_____

_____

_____

⌁ Are you willing to have your own back always and take full responsibility for how you treat yourself in the good times and the bad ? Why or why not? ⌁

_____

_____

_____

♡ Write down what you most need to hear right now. ♡

_____

_____

_____

_____

_____

♡ Channel the kindest, nicest person you know and read that out loud to yourself. ♡

♡ Write mantras out of what you most need to hear, especially ones that fly in the face of whatever thoughts/emotions got you rolling toward self-abuse. ♡

_____

_____

_____

_____

_____

♡ Repeat out loud whenever you are struggling. ♡

♡ Write a list of activities (not food-related) that give you joy. ♡

_____

_____

_____

_____

♡ Go do one of those things today. ♡

·» Not forgiving yourself «·

∾ How is not forgiving yourself serving you? Is it helping you or harming you? ∾

_____

_____

_____

∾ Do you believe you need to forgive yourself? Why or why not? ∾

_____

_____

_____

∾ Are you willing to forgive yourself? Why or why not? ∾

_____

_____

_____

∾ Take a deep breath. ∾
∾ Write a list of events, mistakes, failures, happenings, and the like from your past that you refuse to forgive yourself for. ∾

_____

_____

_____

❧ Take a deep breath. ☙

❧ More space to write things that you refuse to forgive yourself for. ☙

_____

_____

_____

_____

_____

_____

_____

_____

_____

_____

_____

_____

❧ Read through this list and next to each item write the age you were when that particular item occurred. Subtract from your current age. That's how much time you've been imprisoned in unforgiveness. ☙

❧ Take a deep breath. ☙

❧ For each item on your list, ask yourself: Is it possible I just made a mistake, that this was simply an error in judgment? Or I made a decision out of fear, anger, arrogance, loneliness, sadness, and the like? Or maybe I was young and naive? Or maybe, no matter my age, I simply didn't know better and so I didn't do better? ☙

❧ For each item on that list, write an answer to this: What do you need to do to let this go? ❧

_____

_____

_____

_____

_____

_____

_____

_____

❧ Love yourself enough to do whatever it is you need to do to forgive yourself. ❧

❧ Write this: I forgive you. ❧

_____

_____

❧ Write this: I am forgiven. ❧

_____

_____

❧ Look yourself in the eyes in a mirror and say those two phrases aloud to yourself. ❧

❧ Repeat daily for 66 days until they become the story that you believe and so live out in your life. ❧

❧ Are you willing to love yourself enough to forgive yourself over and over and over again, as many times as it takes? Why or why not? ☙

_____

_____

_____

❧ Choose to love yourself enough to forgive yourself because that's how you'll find peace. ☙

⟫ Not forgiving others ⟪

❧ How is not forgiving others serving you? Is it helping you or harming you? ☙

_____

_____

_____

❧ Are you willing to believe you need to forgive others for yourself and your own well-being? Why or why not? ☙

_____

_____

_____

phenomenal

❧ Write a list of people whom you refuse to forgive and what they did or didn't do to you. ☙

_____

_____

_____

_____

_____

_____

_____

_____

_____

❧ Realize and take to heart that people are fallible. ☙

❧ Take a deep breath. ☙

❧ Write an answer to these: Do you really want to exchange your life for chasing after others and traveling in a circle? Or would you rather move on without them in a straight line toward where and who you most want to be? ☙

_____

_____

_____

❧ You be the one to break the cycle, right now. ☙

·» Trying to impress others «·

◌ How is trying to impress others serving you? Is it helping you or harming you? ◌

_____

_____

_____

◌ Write a list of instances when you were trying to impress others. ◌

_____

_____

_____

_____

_____

_____

◌ Take a deep breath. ◌

◌ Why were you trying to impress? What did you hope to gain? ◌

_____

_____

_____

_____

♡ Who was your motivation in those moments when you were trying to impress? ♡

_____

_____

_____

♡ Where was your focus in those moments when you were trying to impress? ♡

_____

_____

_____

♡ Write this: I never need to impress anyone to have worth and value. ♡

_____

_____

_____

♡ Now say that out loud and believe it because your worth and value are innate. ♡

♡ Are you willing to strive to be true to yourself, for your own standards of excellence, and to make yourself fulfilled instead of striving to impress? Why or why not? ♡

_____

_____

_____

·» Trying to save others «·

⊘ How is trying to save others serving you? Is it helping you or harming you? ⊘

_____

_____

_____

⊘ Are you willing to be open to the possibility that all the time, energy, money, and focus you're using turning other people's problems into your own is all the time, energy, money, and focus taken away from you meeting your own goals and dreams? Why or why not? ⊘

_____

_____

_____

⊘ Take a deep breath. ⊘
⊘ Write a list of people whom you're trying to save/whose lives you're trying to fix. ⊘

_____

_____

_____

_____

_____

_____

⊘ For each one, write an answer to this beside their name: Are they capable of saving themselves? ⊘

♡ If the answer is no, then answer this: How can you help them so they can be capable of saving themselves? ♡

_____

_____

_____

_____

_____

_____

_____

♡ In a temporary way and in a supportive role, so they don't become your main focus. ♡

♡ Do you believe you empower others when you make them responsible for their own lives? Why or why not? ♡

_____

_____

_____

♡ Do you believe you empower yourself when you make others responsible for their own lives? Why or why not? ♡

_____

_____

◁ Are you willing to gently but firmly tell others that they need to take the lead on fixing their own problems? Why or why not? ▷

_____

_____

_____

◁ Now you step back and let everyone on your list who is capable (all the yes answers) save themselves. ▷

·" Expecting others to make you happy "·

◁ How is expecting others to make you happy serving you? Is it helping you or harming you? ▷

_____

_____

_____

◁ Do you believe your own happiness is your choice? Why or why not? ▷

_____

_____

_____

◁ Take a deep breath. ▷
◁ Does overeating, starving, purging, and/or abusing food make you genuinely happy? ▷

_____

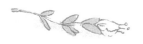 ◁ If not, you can and need to choose differently. ▷

♡ Define for yourself exactly what makes you happy. So write answers to these: What is/was happening in your life when you're at your happiest? What activities make/used to make you feel alive? What do you enjoy doing and/or lights a spark in you? Who do you enjoy being around? Where do you feel most at home? What do you most want to be doing with your life? ♡

_____

_____

_____

_____

_____

_____

_____

_____

_____

_____

_____

_____

_____

_____

♡ Now get busy creating a life around your own answers. ♡

·» Choosing powerlessness over being powerful «·

⊘ How is choosing powerlessness over being powerful serving you? Is it helping you or harming you? ⊙

_____

_____

_____

⊘ Do you believe, at any given moment, you can choose to either be powerless or be powerful but not both at the same time? Why or why not? ⊙

_____

_____

_____

⊘ Take a deep breath. ⊙
⊘ Look at the situation you currently find yourself in and write a list of everything that's not the way you want it to be. ⊙

_____

_____

_____

_____

_____

_____

_____

☙ Take a deep breath. ❧
☙ More space to write what's not the way you want it to be. ❧

♡ For each item on the list you just wrote, answer these: What choices do you need to make that will improve your situation? What choices are best for you? What choices will move you in the direction that you want to go? ♡

_____

_____

_____

_____

_____

_____

_____

_____

_____

_____

_____

_____

_____

_____

_____

♡ Write some strength to yourself. What do you most need to hear right now? ♡

_____

_____

_____

_____

♡ Speak it out loud. ♡
♡ Now get busy making choices and taking actions that are best for you. ♡

·» Panic, despair, and worry «·

♡ How is panicking serving you? Is it helping you or harming you? ♡

_____

_____

_____

♡ Take a deep breath. ♡
♡ Write a list of instances when you made decisions while panicking. ♡

_____

_____

_____

_____

_____

⊲ How did each of those decisions turn out? ⊳

_____

_____

_____

_____

_____

⊲ Are you willing, from now on, to take a step back from a situation if at all possible and wait to make a decision? Why or why not? ⊳

_____

_____

_____

⊲ How is despair serving you? Is it helping you or harming you? ⊳

_____

_____

_____

tenacious

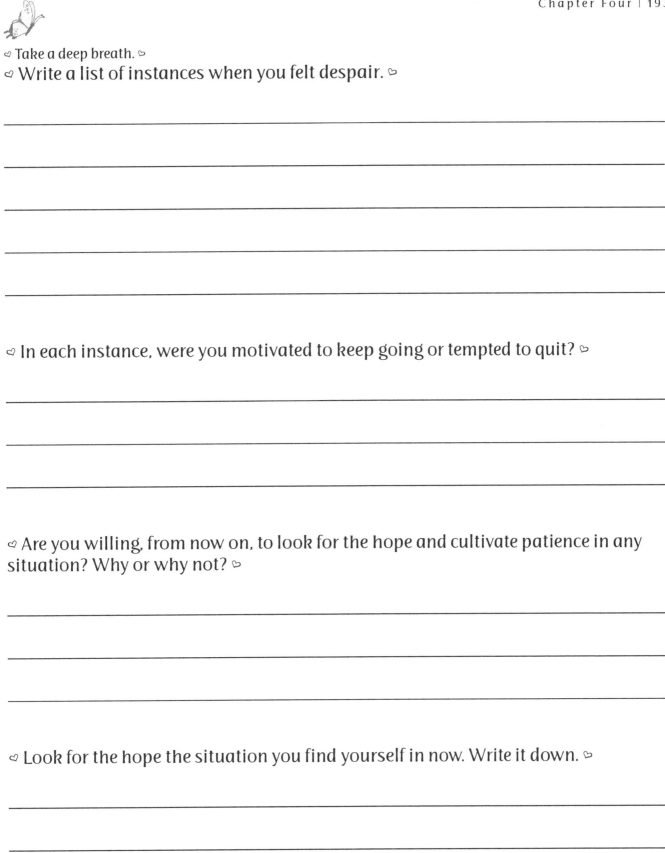

ↂ Take a deep breath. ↂ
ↂ Write a list of instances when you felt despair. ↂ

_____

_____

_____

_____

ↂ In each instance, were you motivated to keep going or tempted to quit? ↂ

_____

_____

_____

ↂ Are you willing, from now on, to look for the hope and cultivate patience in any situation? Why or why not? ↂ

_____

_____

_____

ↂ Look for the hope the situation you find yourself in now. Write it down. ↂ

_____

_____

_____

ↂ Now hang on to that hope. ↂ

❥ How is worry serving you? Is it helping you or harming you? ❦

_____

_____

_____

❥ Take a deep breath. ❦
❥ Write a list of instances when you worried about the outcome. ❦

_____

_____

_____

_____

❥ In each instance, did your worrying change the outcome at all? If so, how? ❦

_____

_____

❥ Write a list of choices you can make and actions you can take that will fix whatever situation it is that you're worrying about. ❦

_____

_____

_____

❥ Now take action to fix your situation. ❦

❧ Are you willing to believe that you're strong enough to handle anything that life hands you? Why or why not? ☙

_____

_____

_____

❧ Choose to believe that you are strong enough to handle life as it comes. ☙

·›› Things that don't belong to you and/or aren't about you ‹‹·

❧ How is holding on to things that don't belong to you and/or aren't about you serving you? Is it helping you or harming you? ☙

_____

_____

_____

❧ Take a deep breath. ☙
❧ Write an inventory of things inside yourself that you may be struggling with and/or that don't feel true to you. ☙

_____

_____

_____

_____

_____

_____

⨀ Take a deep breath. ⨀

⨀ More space to write an inventory of things that don't feel true to you. ⨀

_____

_____

_____

_____

_____

_____

_____

_____

_____

_____

_____

_____

_____

⨀ Take a deep breath. ⨀

⨀ For each item, ask: Is this true for me? Do I actually believe this? Do I want to believe this? Who does this actually belong to? Or for blame/responsibility: Is this actually my doing? ⨀

᪥ What do you need to do for yourself to reject/release all those things that don't belong to you? ᪥

_____

_____

_____

_____

᪥ Don't wait. Do it now. ᪥
᪥ Then step around them and keep on going. ᪥

⠺ Getting in your own way ⠺

᪥ How is getting in your own way serving you? Is it helping you or harming you? ᪥
᪥ List any benefits you gain by being overweight and/or abusing food. ᪥

_____

_____

_____

᪥ Go back to pages 142–143 and reread your answers as to what you truly believe about yourself. ᪥
᪥ Write a list of instances (both big crossroad-type moments and itty-bitty moments) in your life where you regret the choice you made, especially if that choice took you further away from what you wanted. ᪥

_____

_____

_____

❧ Take a deep breath. ☙

❧ More space to write a list where you regret the choice you made. ☙

_____

_____

_____

_____

_____

_____

❧ Take a deep breath and listen for your intuition. ☙

❧ Write an answer to this: Why did you sabotage yourself in each of those moments? ☙

_____

_____

_____

_____

_____

_____

_____

❧ Hint: the answer likely has something to do with fear. ☙

ᴏ Read through the answers you just wrote and find the common thread between them. Write it down. ᴏ

_____

_____

_____

_____

ᴏ That thread is likely your biggest fear and the major reason that you keep getting in your own way. ᴏ

ᴏ Are you willing to trust your intuition, let it guide you, and do what it tells you even if that scares you? Why or why not? ᴏ

_____

_____

_____

ᴏ Listen for your intuition and write down what it's telling you that you need to do to move forward in your life. ᴏ

_____

_____

_____

_____

ᴏ Take a deep breath. ᴏ
ᴏ Now take that action(s) today. ᴏ

·» Trying to control «·

♡ How is trying to control serving you? Is it helping you or harming you? ♡

_____

_____

_____

♡ Take a deep breath. ♡
♡ Write a list of people, situations, outcomes, etc. that you are trying to control. ♡

_____

_____

_____

_____

_____

_____

_____

_____

♡ How has trying to control those things worked out for you? ♡

_____

_____

_____

⏃ What has been your reaction when things didn't work out like you'd wanted? ⏂

_____

_____

_____

⏃ Are you willing to believe that control is just an illusion? Why or why not? ⏂

_____

_____

_____

⏃ Are you willing to honor yourself by following your own passions and cultivating your own gifts and talents? Why or why not? ⏂

_____

_____

_____

⏃ Are you willing to respect yourself by making clear boundaries and defending them? Why or why not? ⏂

_____

_____

_____

⌒ Are you willing to determine what you want for your life because it deeply matters to you? Why or why not? ⌒

_____

_____

_____

⌒ Are you willing to keep moving forward without delay? Why or why not? ⌒

_____

_____

_____

⌒ Are you willing to believe without a doubt that life is rigged in your favor? Why or why not? ⌒

_____

_____

_____

⌒ Are you willing to believe without a doubt that there is a lesson in everything that happens to you and that lesson is a gift to you? Why or why not? ⌒

_____

_____

_____

⌒ You are strong enough and capable enough to get through everything without abusing food for relief. ⌒

·» **This is a practice and a process** «·

⊲ What worked for you during this chapter? What didn't? ⊳

_____

_____

_____

_____

_____

_____

⊲ Always, always, always find what works for you and do that. ⊳
⊲ You have permission to let go, right now, of anything that doesn't work for you. ⊳

⊲ Write a list of things you've learned from your mistakes. ⊳

_____

_____

_____

_____

⊲ Learn what you can, come at it again from a wiser perspective, then move on. ⊳
⊲ Remember: every mistake is simply a brand new chance to do it better the next time. ⊳

Chapter Five!

·» The most important thing you may ever learn about weight loss «·

Are you willing to believe that clinging to all those people, places, and/or things that no longer serve you is actually sucking the life out of you? Why or why not?

_____

_____

_____

Write an instance when you clung to a person, place, or thing and how that turned out for you in the end.

_____

_____

_____

_____

Are you willing to believe that excising your vampires is the single most important thing you can do not only for your weight loss but also for your happiness in general? Why or why not?

_____

_____

_____

·» **Your body will tell you everything you need to know** «·

♡ Are you willing to believe that your intuition will tell you what your vampires are, how to get rid of them, and most importantly when it's time to move on without them? Why or why not? ♡

_____

_____

_____

♡ What are you afraid is going to happen to you when you let go of your vampires? ♡

_____

_____

_____

♡ Write this: No one is coming to fix it. I must save myself. ♡

_____

_____

♡ What cues has your body given you when you've been in contact with a vampire or even just thinking about one? ♡

_____

_____

_____

♡ Are you willing to trust your body and listen to how it feels and reacts? Why or why not? ♡

_____

_____

_____

·» People you're going to have to banish from your life «·

♡ Are you willing to believe that some people (even people you may love) are vampires for you? Why or why not? ♡

_____

_____

_____

♡ Are you willing to pay attention to a person's behavior, not make excuses for them, and see them for who they really are the first time? Why or why not? ♡

_____

_____

_____

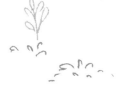

♡ Three easy ways to spot a vampire. ♡

♡ If they lie to you (little white lies included). ♡

♡ If they are in any way abusive (physically, verbally, sexually, mentally/emotionally) to you. ♡

♡ If you react to anyone by abusing food and/or some other substance(s)/behavior(s) before, during, and/or after you're with them just to tolerate the encounter. ♡

❧ Write a list of family members that are vampires for you. ☙

_____

_____

_____

_____

❧ Write a list of work-related people that are vampires for you. ☙

_____

_____

_____

_____

❧ Write a list of "friends" that are vampires for you. ☙

_____

_____

_____

_____

_____

❧ Write a list of significant others that are vampires for you. ❧

_____

_____

_____

_____

_____

❧ Write a list of acquaintances and strangers that are vampires for you. ❧

_____

_____

_____

_____

_____

❧ Are you willing to limit your time with and/or cut out of your life entirely all the people you've listed above? Why or why not? ❧

_____

_____

_____

_____

_____

_____

♡ Write a list of vampire people, if any, with whom you have an interest in salvaging the relationship. ♡

_____

_____

_____

_____

♡ Pick the person listed above whose relationship means the most to you. Write a letter to them. What do you most need them to hear? Be honest. ♡

_____

_____

_____

_____

_____

_____

_____

_____

_____

_____

♡ This is for you to heal yourself. If you want to heal the relationship, share this letter with them. ♡

⊄ Are you willing to let them go if you cannot make the relationship a healthy one? Why or why not? ⊅

_____

_____

_____

⊄ You always have permission to protect yourself from people who suck the life out of you. ⊅
⊄ Remember: it's your life you're working to save. ⊅

⊄ Are you willing to defend your own boundaries? Why or why not? ⊅

_____

_____

_____

⊄ Write a list of activities that fulfill and nourish you. ⊅

_____

_____

_____

_____

_____

_____

⊄ Do one or more of those activities before and after encounters with people who are vampires for you. ⊅
⊄ You are worth taking excellent care of yourself. ⊅

◌ Have you been a vampire with life-sucking behavior toward others? If so, how? ◌

_____

_____

_____

◌ Are you willing to stand on your own two feet and stop searching for anyone else to be your life source? Why or why not? ◌

_____

_____

_____

◌ Remember: no one is coming to fix it. ◌

·» Places you're going to have to banish from your life «·

◌ Are you willing to believe some places are vampires for you? Why or why not? ◌

_____

_____

_____

◌ Are you willing to pay attention to how your body feels when you're in a particular place and heed any warnings it may be giving you? Why or why not? ◌

_____

_____

_____

୯ Write a list of places that you know are vampires for you. ಲ

_____

_____

_____

_____

_____

୯ Write a list of reasons why you go to or stay in those vampire places. ಲ

_____

_____

_____

_____

_____

୯ Are you willing to honor and respect yourself by leaving or avoiding a place that drains the life from you? Why or why not? ಲ

_____

_____

_____

spectacular

❧ Do you live in a vampire place? If so, what specifically is sucking the life out of you? ☙

_____

_____

_____

_____

_____

❧ What can you do to change that place and make it more nourishing for you? ☙

_____

_____

_____

_____

_____

❧ Take action (even small) to change where you live today. ☙

❧ Do you work in a vampire place? If so, what specifically is sucking the life out of you? ☙

_____

_____

_____

_____

_____

◁ What can you do to change that place and make it more nourishing for you? ▷

_____

_____

_____

_____

_____

◁ Take action (even small) to change where you work today. ▷

◁ Do you visit a vampire place? If so, what specifically is sucking the life out of you? ▷

_____

_____

_____

_____

◁ Why do you keep visiting that place? ▷

_____

_____

_____

_____

_____

❧ If you're unable to stop visiting that place, what can you do to change that place and make it more nourishing for you? ❧

_____

_____

_____

_____

❧ Take action (even small) to change where you visit today. ❧

❧ Do you play in a vampire place? If so, what specifically is sucking the life out of you? ❧

_____

_____

_____

_____

❧ What can you do to change that place and make it more nourishing for you? ❧

_____

_____

_____

_____

❧ Take action (even small) to change where you play today. ❧

❧ Do you create in a vampire place? If so, what specifically is sucking the life out of you? ❧

_____

_____

_____

_____

_____

❧ What can you do to change that place and make it more nourishing for you? ❧

_____

_____

_____

_____

❧ Take action (even small) to change where you create today. ❧

❧ Are you willing to respect yourself by meeting your actual preferences, wants, and needs? Why or why not? ❧

_____

_____

_____

❧ Write a list of places that make you happy and fulfilled when you go there. ☙

_____

_____

_____

_____

❧ Are you willing to choose to go those places that make you happier and more fulfilled instead of places that suck the life out of you? Why or why not? ☙

_____

_____

_____

❧ Write a list of excuses you're using to remain in vampire places. ☙

_____

_____

_____

❧ Are you willing to stop making excuses and instead relocate, redecorate, and/or whatever it is you need to do to create places that nourish you? Why or why not? ☙

_____

_____

❧ Remember: the choice is always up to you. ☙

·» Thoughts and beliefs you're going to have to banish from your life «·

♡ Are you willing to believe some thoughts and beliefs are vampires for you? Why or why not? ♡

_____

_____

_____

♡ Do you agree that you are what you believe you are and you will live out what you believe? Why or why not? ♡

_____

_____

_____

♡ Finish this sentence: I am . . . ♡

_____

_____

_____

♡ Are you willing to change what you believe, especially those beliefs that are vampires for you? Why or why not? ♡

_____

_____

_____

♡ Are you willing to remake yourself? Are you willing to become somebody new? Why or why not? ♡

_____

_____

_____

♡ Let your intuition guide you and write a list of thoughts/beliefs that you know are vampires for you. ♡

_____

_____

_____

_____

_____

_____

_____

♡ Write a list of reasons why you allow those thoughts/beliefs to remain in your head. ♡

_____

_____

_____

_____

❧ Write a list of labels that are vampires for you. ☙

_____

_____

_____

_____

_____

_____

_____

❧ For each one, ask: Is this true? Do I want it to be true for me? ☙
❧ Reject any and all beliefs that drain you. That choice is always yours. ☙

❧ Write what you would rather think/believe about yourself instead. ☙

_____

_____

_____

_____

_____

_____

_____

❧ What is true for you? What beliefs will help you move forward and grow? ☙
❧ Repeat, repeat, repeat those new thoughts and take action as if they are already true. ☙

❧ Write a list of judgments that are vampires for you. ❧

_____

_____

_____

_____

_____

_____

_____

❧ For each one, ask: Is this true? Do I want it to be true for me? ❧
❧ Reject any and all beliefs that drain you. That choice is always yours. ❧

❧ Write what you would rather think/believe about yourself instead. ❧

_____

_____

_____

_____

_____

_____

❧ What is true for you? What beliefs will help you move forward and grow? ❧
❧ Repeat, repeat, repeat those new thoughts and take action as if they are already true. ❧

❧ Write a list of things you were taught that are vampires for you. ❧

_____

_____

_____

_____

_____

_____

_____

❧ For each one, ask: Is this true? Do I want it to be true for me? ❧
❧ Reject any and all beliefs that drain you. That choice is always yours. ❧

❧ Write what you would rather think/believe about yourself instead. ❧

_____

_____

_____

_____

_____

_____

_____

❧ What is true for you? What beliefs will help you move forward and grow? ❧
❧ Repeat, repeat, repeat those new thoughts and take action as if they are already true. ❧

⌂ Write a list of things you were told or overheard that are vampires for you. ⌂

_____

_____

_____

_____

_____

_____

⌂ For each one, ask: Is this true? Do I want it to be true for me? ⌂
⌂ Reject any and all beliefs that drain you. That choice is always yours. ⌂

⌂ Write what you would rather think/believe about yourself instead. ⌂

_____

_____

_____

_____

_____

_____

⌂ What is true for you? What beliefs will help you move forward and grow? ⌂
⌂ Repeat, repeat, repeat those new thoughts and take action as if they are already true. ⌂

◌ Write a list of things you chose (and still choose) to believe that are vampires for you. ◌

_____

_____

_____

_____

_____

_____

◌ For each one, ask: Is this true? Do I want it to be true for me? ◌
◌ Reject any and all beliefs that drain you. That choice is always yours. ◌

◌ Write what you would rather think/believe about yourself instead. ◌

_____

_____

_____

_____

_____

_____

◌ What is true for you? What beliefs will help you move forward and grow? ◌
◌ Repeat, repeat, repeat those new thoughts and take action as if they are already true. ◌

·» Addictions you're going to have to banish from your life «·

♡ Are you willing to believe that addictions are vampires for you? Why or why not? ♡

_____

_____

_____

♡ Do you believe addicted people have a disease or a choice? Why? ♡

_____

_____

_____

♡ Are you willing to make the changes you need to make to stop any addiction(s) you may have and heal yourself of its cause? Why or why not? ♡

_____

_____

_____

♡ Remember: no one is coming to fix it. ♡

♡ Are you willing to pay attention to how your body feels when you're doing any particular activity and heed any warnings it may be giving you? Why or why not? ♡

_____

_____

_____

ᧄ Write how food is currently a vampire for you. ᧄ

_____

_____

_____

_____

_____

ᧄ Write down how that addiction started. ᧄ

_____

_____

_____

_____

ᧄ Write down why you're abusing food. What are you hoping to gain? ᧄ

_____

_____

_____

_____

_____

⊘ Write how any other substances (if applicable) are currently a vampire for you. ⊘

_____

_____

_____

_____

_____

⊘ Write down how that addiction started. ⊘

_____

_____

_____

_____

⊘ Write down why you're abusing those substances. What are you hoping to gain? ⊘

_____

_____

_____

_____

❧ Write how any people/relationships (if applicable) are currently a vampire for you. ☙

_____

_____

_____

_____

_____

❧ Write down how that addiction started. ☙

_____

_____

_____

_____

❧ Write down why you're abusing those relationships. What are you hoping to gain? ☙

_____

_____

_____

_____

♥ Write how any other behaviors (if applicable) are currently a vampire for you. ♥

_____

_____

_____

_____

_____

♥ Write down how that addiction started. ♥

_____

_____

_____

_____

_____

♥ Write down why you're abusing those behaviors. What are you hoping to gain? ♥

_____

_____

_____

_____

_____

♡ Write down anything else you use to escape your life (which means it's a vampire for you). ♡

_____

_____

_____

_____

_____

♡ Write down how that addiction started. ♡

_____

_____

_____

_____

♡ Write down why you're abusing those things. What are you hoping to gain? ♡

_____

_____

_____

_____

_____

✑ Write this: The real me is the only person worth being in the world. ✑

_____

_____

✑ Write this: I don't owe the world my life. ✑

_____

✑ Write this: I owe it to myself to show up in the world as the real me. ✑

_____

_____

✑ Write this: The real me is enough as-is. The real me is valuable as-is. ✑

_____

_____

✑ Write this: My passions, gifts, and talents matter because I matter. ✑

_____

_____

✑ Write this: I am worth the effort. ✑

_____

✑ Write this: No one is coming to fix it. ✑

_____

✑ Repeat those phrases until they become the story that you believe and so live out in your life. ✑

❧ Are you willing to give yourself permission to do whatever you need to do to reach your goal of being healthy and feeling whole again? Why or why not? ☙

_____

_____

_____

❧ Write yourself a permission slip (and a promise to yourself) right now. ☙
❧ Example: I have permission and will do whatever I need to do to reach my goal of being healthy and feeling whole again. Then sign your name and date. ☙

_____

_____

_____

_____

Name:_____**Date:**_____

❧ So honor yourself and keep your word to yourself. ☙
❧ You be actively involved and determined in your own healing. ☙

❧ Speak strength to yourself and write the words you most need to hear right now. ☙

_____

_____

_____

_____

_____

☙ Space to write down the truth about anyone/anything else that needs to be addressed. ❧
☙ This is just for you so be honest. Lay it all out so you can see exactly what you're dealing with. ❧

_____

_____

_____

_____

_____

_____

_____

_____

_____

_____

_____

_____

_____

_____

_____

_____

❧ Write a list of people whom you trust to talk to about overcoming any addiction(s). ☙

_____

_____

_____

❧ Pick one and tell them the truth about the addiction(s) you're determined to overcome. ☙

❧ What do you most need to help you? ☙

_____

_____

_____

❧ Take action now and do whatever you need to do to take care of yourself. ☙

❧ Are you willing to be actively involved and determined in your own healing? Why or why not? ☙

_____

_____

_____

❧ Remember: no one is coming to fix it. ☙

❧ Are you willing to persevere? Why or why not? ☙

_____

_____

_____

❧ Don't stop until you're free. ☙

·» Armor you're going to have to banish from your life «·

♡ Are you willing to believe armor is a vampire for you? Why or why not? ♡

_____

_____

_____

♡ Are you willing to believe armor is all about hiding the real you and keeping that real you hidden? Why or why not? ♡

_____

_____

_____

♡ Are you willing to believe that when you use armor, you're the one who ends up encased in a shell? Why or why not? ♡

_____

_____

_____

♡ Armor doesn't let you out. ♡

♡ Are you willing to believe armor is just an illusion of safety? Why or why not? ♡

_____

_____

_____

♡ Armor takes something from you. ♡

♡ Write a list of reactions from your mind and body that signal you're using armor. ♡

_____

_____

_____

_____

_____

_____

♡ So do yourself a kindness and listen to your intuition. ♡

♡ Write down how physical distance (if applicable) is a vampire for you. ♡

_____

_____

_____

_____

_____

♡ Write a permission slip and give yourself permission to be yourself. ♡

_____

_____

_____

_____

♡ You free yourself by being yourself. ♡
♡ There's only one life you can really save; that's your own. ♡

♡ Write down how mental distance (if applicable) is a vampire for you. ♡

_____

_____

_____

_____

♡ Write a permission slip and give yourself permission to be yourself. ♡

_____

_____

_____

_____

♡ You free yourself by being yourself. ♡
♡ There's only one life you can really save; that's your own. ♡

♡ Write down how busyness (if applicable) is a vampire for you. ♡

_____

_____

_____

_____

❧ Write a permission slip and give yourself permission to be yourself. ❧

_____

_____

_____

_____

❧ You free yourself by being yourself. ❧
❧ There's only one life you can really save; that's your own. ❧

❧ Write down how material things (if applicable) are a vampire for you. ❧

_____

_____

_____

_____

❧ Write a permission slip and give yourself permission to be yourself. ❧

_____

_____

_____

_____

❧ You free yourself by being yourself. ❧
❧ There's only one life you can really save; that's your own. ❧

❧ Write down how saying no to opportunities (if applicable) is a vampire for you. ☙

_____

_____

_____

_____

_____

❧ Write a permission slip and give yourself permission to be yourself. ☙

_____

_____

_____

_____

❧ You free yourself by being yourself. ☙
❧ There's only one life you can really save; that's your own. ☙

❧ Are you willing to say yes? Why or why not? ☙

_____

_____

_____

❧ Remember: the moment you say no, your journey down that particular path ends. ☙

♡ Write a list of things you want to say yes to. ♡

_____

_____

_____

_____

_____

_____

_____

♡ Write this: I am strong enough as myself to handle whatever comes my way. ♡

_____

_____

_____

♡ Now look yourself in the eyes in a mirror and repeat that phrase aloud. ♡

♡ Write this: I'm living my life for me. ♡

_____

_____

♡ Hold that in your heart and keep it at the top of your mind every time you make a choice. ♡

♡ Are you willing to show up without your armor? Why or why not? ♡

_____

_____

_____

♡ Are you willing to relax into the process? Why or why not? ♡

_____

_____

_____

♡ Take a deep breath in through your nose, hold it three seconds, let it out slowly through your mouth. ♡

♡ Write this: I cannot rise above until I let go of the stuff that holds me down. ♡

_____

_____

♡ Write this: I free myself by being myself. ♡

_____

_____

♡ Write this: There's only one life I can really save, and that's my own. ♡

_____

_____

 ♡ Now go pursue your own gifts, talents, passions, wants, hopes, and/or dreams. ♡

·» This is a practice and a process «·

◁ **What worked for you during this chapter? What didn't?** ▷

_____

_____

_____

_____

_____

_____

◁ Always, always, always find what works for you and do that. ▷
◁ You have permission to let go, right now, of anything that doesn't work for you. ▷

◁ **Write a list of things you've learned from your mistakes.** ▷

_____

_____

_____

_____

_____

◁ Learn what you can, come at it again from a wiser perspective, then move on. ▷
◁ Remember: every mistake is simply a brand new chance to do it better the next time. ▷

·» Notes or doodles «·

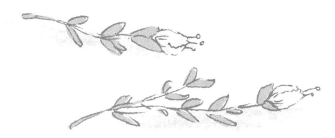

Chapter Six!

·» You are alive for a reason «·

◁ Are you willing to believe that you are alive for a reason? Why or why not? ▷

_____

_____

_____

◁ Are you willing to believe that you have both a gift (or more than one) and a purpose? Why or why not? ▷

_____

_____

_____

◁ Write an instance when you experienced incongruence—knowing you are one kind of person but denying it while attempting to pass yourself off as another—and how that made you feel. ▷

_____

_____

_____

_____

◌ Are you willing to find your gift? Why or why not? ◌

_____

_____

_____

◌ Are you willing to believe If you do nothing else with your life other than find your gift and share it with others, you'll have done enough? Why or why not? ◌

_____

_____

_____

◌ Write this: I am only responsible for saving my own life. ◌

_____

_____

◌ Write this: I am strong. I am a survivor. I don't need anyone or anything else to make me whole. ◌

_____

_____

_____

◌ Now take those phrases to heart and believe them. ◌

How have you been pretending that you're someone else (the self or selves that don't ring true to you)?

_____

_____

_____

_____

_____

Do you like the real you? Why or why not?

_____

_____

_____

·» So stop hiding your light «·

Are you willing to believe that shining your own light is when you're at your most powerful? Why or why not?

_____

_____

_____

talented

❧ Write a list of gifts, talents, and passions that you know you have. ☙

_____

_____

_____

_____

_____

❧ Are you willing to actively seek out and cultivate your gifts, talents, and passions and help them grow? Why or why not? ☙

_____

_____

_____

❧ Are you willing to make yourself your motivation to shine your gifts, talents, and passions (to bring yourself fulfillment and joy as well as to give your life deeper meaning)? Why or why not? ☙

_____

_____

_____

❧ How can you shine your gifts, talents, and passions by sharing them with others? ☙

_____

_____

_____

✎ Are you willing to shine your gifts, talents, and passions by sharing them with others? Why or why not? ✎

_____

_____

_____

✎ What constraints have you put on doing what you're brilliant at? ✎

_____

_____

_____

_____

_____

_____

✎ Are you willing to let yourself do what you're brilliant at, wholeheartedly and without constraints? Why or why not? ✎

_____

_____

_____

✎ Write this: Hiding my light serves no one, least of all myself. ✎

_____

_____

◌ Why do you think you're in so much pain? Why do you think you're trying to numb yourself? Why do you think the cycle of abusing substances/behaviors continues over and over and over again? ◌

_____

_____

_____

_____

_____

_____

_____

◌ Do you believe when you dim your own light and hide the real you, you cause a rift (hole/wound) inside yourself? Why or why not? ◌

_____

_____

_____

◌ Are you willing to believe it's the rift (the being at constant odds with yourself, the incongruence) that's tearing you apart and fueling the numbing activities you do? Why or why not? ◌

_____

_____

_____

◌ Write this: When I fail to shine my own light, I shrink my life down to the size and shape of those who would dim me and I never get to realize my own potential. ◌

_____

_____

_____

_____

◌ Now take that to heart and believe it because it's true. ◌

·» You may choose to hide your light because you're afraid «·

◌ What are you afraid will happen to you if you shine your light? ◌

_____

_____

_____

_____

◌ Why are you afraid that will happen? ◌

_____

_____

_____

❧ Write an instance when you dimmed yourself to the level of those around you so you could blend in. ☙

_____

_____

_____

_____

❧ Now write how that made you feel. ☙

_____

_____

_____

_____

⟐ You may choose to hide your light because you didn't receive what you hoped you would ⟐

❧ Have you ever quit pursuing your gifts, talents, and passions because they didn't earn you something tangible in the end? If so, write which one(s). ☙

_____

_____

_____

_____

_____

❧ What were you hoping to receive and in what time frame? ☙

_____

_____

_____

❧ Are you willing to make your well-being your sole motivation and let go of the outcome so you can heal? Why or why not? ☙

_____

_____

_____

·» You may choose to hide your light because you are plagued by self-doubt «·

❧ Do you trust yourself to know what shines a light in you? Why or why not? ☙

_____

_____

_____

❧ Do you trust your intuition to guide you toward your gifts, talents, and/or passions? Why or why not? ☙

_____

_____

_____

Do you trust your ability to achieve your own hopes, wants, dreams, and/or desires? Why or why not?

_____

_____

_____

Do you believe you are worthy and deserving of doing what shines a light in you? Why or why not?

_____

_____

_____

Are you willing to believe that the urge to shine your light versus the act of stopping yourself from doing it is at the heart of that rift we've been talking about? Why or why not?

_____

_____

_____

·» You may choose to hide your light because your definition of success does not include using your gifts, talents, and passions «·

Go back to page 164 and read your definition of success. Now answer this: Does that definition include doing what shines a light in you? If not, why not?

_____

_____

☙ Now write a definition of success that includes your gifts, talents, and passions. ☚

_____

_____

_____

_____

_____

_____

_____

_____

_____

_____

_____

**»» You may choose to hide your light because you put
the needs of others before your own ««**

☙ Are you willing to believe that using your gifts, talents, and passions is a need?
Why or why not? ☚

_____

_____

_____

☙ These are needs: the sense that you have a purpose in the world, the belief that you have unique
gifts and talents, and being creative to bring yourself fulfillment and happiness. ☚

❧ Do you want to spend your time abusing substances/behaviors or do you want to spend it fulfilling yourself? ❧

_____

_____

_____

❧ Remember: you're exchanging your life for what you choose to do with your time. ❧

❧ Write your priority list. Now write your name at the very top of that list. ❧

_____

_____

_____

_____

_____

_____

_____

_____

_____

_____

_____

·» A quick exercise to excavate the real you «·

ღ What makes me feel the most alive. ღ | ღ Why I don't do it. ღ

·» So how do you let go of hiding your light «·

♡ Write this: I choose to believe my gifts, talents, and passions matter deeply to me. ♡

_____

_____

♡ Write this: I choose to believe that actively pursuing my gifts, talents, and passions also deeply matters to me. ♡

_____

_____

_____

♡ Choose to believe those two statements every day. ♡

♡ Say these aloud: Hiding my light only widens that rift inside me. Hiding my light is part of the reason I continue abusing food to cope with the pain. Every time I hide my light, I betray myself. Now write any reaction you may have. ♡

_____

_____

_____

♡ Write a permission slip (now and as often as necessary) to let your light shine bright. ♡

_____

_____

_____

·» A seven-step plan to get you to the life you most want «·

·» Step One «·
·» Discover your gifts, talents, and passions «·

◌ What is your head belief? ◌

_____

_____

_____

◌ What is your heart belief? ◌

_____

_____

_____

◌ Are you willing to listen to your life? Why or why not?

_____

_____

_____

intelligent

·» Step 1A: Listen to your life «·

♡ Go back to page 256 and read what makes you feel the most alive. Now add any other activities that you naturally gravitate toward, have an interest in (even a little), and/or make you feel happy and in the present moment. ♡

_____

_____

_____

_____

_____

_____

_____

♡ Describe your perfect day. ♡

_____

_____

_____

_____

_____

_____

_____

❧ Look back at your history. Write what you loved to do when you were a kid, what you most wanted to be when you grew up. ☙

_____

_____

_____

_____

_____

_____

_____

❧ Add anything (and everything) you would love to do if only it weren't for the fear. ☙

_____

_____

_____

_____

_____

_____

_____

·» Step 1B: Pay attention «·
 Do this activity over a period of days/weeks/months.

 Be aware of your own day-to-day life. What piques your interest/makes you lose track of time/causes a little spark to flare inside you when you see, hear, smell, feel, and/or touch it?

_____

_____

_____

_____

_____

_____

_____

_____

_____

_____

_____

_____

_____

_____

·» Step 1C: Find what makes you come alive by finding out what doesn't «·
◁ Do this activity over a period of days/weeks/months. ▷

◁ Pay attention to what you dislike, including activities, people, lifestyle, and/or anything that leaves you feeling drained. ▷

_____

_____

_____

_____

_____

_____

_____

_____

_____

_____

_____

_____

_____

_____

_____

_____

·» Step 1D: Narrow your focus «·

◌ Refer back to pages 256, 259–260 (your answers for excavating the real you and Step 1A of what makes you feel the most alive) and write down the ONE you're most drawn to. ◌

_____

◌ With that ONE thing you love in mind, answer this: What specifically matters to you in that thing? Write the first answers that come to you (so no overthinking or editing). ◌

_____

_____

_____

_____

_____

_____

_____

_____

_____

_____

_____

◌ Be as specific as possible so your answer is tailored just for you. ◌

·» Step 1E: Trust yourself «·

☙ Are you willing to be open to whatever answers come up in you? Why or why not? ❧

_____

_____

_____

☙ Remember: self-trust is the first secret of success. ❧

☙ Write this: I have been with me for my entire life. I know myself better than anyone else. ❧

_____

_____

_____

☙ Write this: I can trust myself. ❧

_____

☙ Take those phrases to heart because they are true. ❧

·» Step 1F: Let go of outside expectations «·

☙ Are you willing to believe that the only thing that's important in discovering who you are is what truly and deeply matters to you? Why or why not? ❧

_____

_____

_____

❤ Write this: I choose to do what I do, with every action I take and every choice I make, to save my own life. ❧

_____

_____

_____

❤ Write this: I will give myself unlimited tries. ❧

_____

_____

❤ Write this: I will forgive myself as many times as it takes. ❧

_____

_____

❤ Honor those phrases because you need to do them to heal. ❧
❤ Honor yourself by keeping your word to yourself. ❧

⁖⟫ Step 1G: Take baby steps if that makes it easier for you ⟪⁖
❤ Start with the ONE activity you chose on page 263 (Narrow your focus).
With that in mind, answer these questions. ❧

❤ Are you willing to take the pressure off and just let yourself experiment? Why or why not? ❧

_____

_____

❤ Are you willing to keep going even if you don't have immediate results? Why or why not? ❤

_____

_____

_____

❤ Are you willing to be open to letting yourself, and what makes you come alive, unfold and grow? Why or why not? ❤

_____

_____

_____

❤ Write this: It's okay to grow slowly. ❤

_____

❤ Take that to heart because it's true. ❤
❤ Now stick with that ONE activity for a time and see where it leads. ❤

·» Step 1H: Hang on to hope and keep on going «·

❤ Are you willing to see what you've started through all the way to the end? Why or why not? ❤

_____

_____

_____

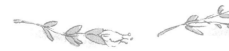
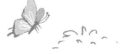

♂ Write this: I will have faith in myself. ♀

_____

♂ Write this: I will hang on to hope. ♀

_____

♂ Write this: I will not stop until I discover what makes me come alive. ♀

_____

_____

♂ Write this: Then I will go do it. ♀

_____

♂ Now honor and respect yourself and do all those things you just promised yourself. ♀

·» Step 11: If you still don't know, try this «·

♂ Take the Survey of Character Strengths online. Write a list of your strengths here. ♀

_____

_____

_____

_____

_____

♂ Now accentuate and nourish those. ♀

·» Step Two «·
·» Define your deepest hopes and desires «·

◌ Read through your definition of success on pages 164 and 254. Now add anything else here to define what a successful life looks like to you. ◌

◌ This is about what you most want for your life, what deeply matters to you. ◌

_____

_____

_____

_____

_____

_____

_____

_____

_____

_____

_____

_____

_____

_____

_____

❧ How can your gifts, talents, and passions help you realize your deepest hopes and desires? ❧

_____

_____

_____

_____

_____

❧ How can you incorporate your gifts, talents, and passions into your life so you can do more of them every day? ❧

_____

_____

_____

_____

_____

❧ Write this: I am worth having my deepest hopes and desires. ❧

_____

_____

_____

  ❧ Now repeat, repeat, repeat that to yourself because it is true. ❧

·» Step 2A: Open yourself up to possibility «·

ᔆ Will you choose to be open and willing? Why or why not? ᔆ

_____

_____

_____

ᔆ Just what if you could have all your hopes and desires come true? How would you feel about your life then? ᔆ

_____

_____

_____

ᔆ What if you could have/be/do/say what makes you feel the most alive? How would you feel about your life then? ᔆ

_____

_____

_____

ᔆ What if every day you woke up excited about your life, happy to have another day to pursue what you love, curious to see what amazing thing is going to happen next? How would you feel about your life then? ᔆ

_____

_____

_____

⊲ Write this: I'm possible. ⊳

_____

⊲ Remember: the only difference between impossible and I'm possible is commitment. ⊳

⊲ What if you truly believed in "I'm possible" no matter what? How would you feel about your life then? ⊳

_____

_____

_____

⊲ Remember: you create the life you're living. ⊳
⊲ If you don't like the path you're on, simply choose differently. ⊳

·» Step 2B: Let your fear point you in the right direction «·

⊲ If you weren't afraid, what would you most want to have/be/do/say? ⊳

_____

_____

_____

_____

_____

_____

_____

⊲ If fear didn't stop you, where would you most want to go from here? ⊳

_____

_____

_____

_____

_____

_____

_____

_____

_____

⊲ Write this: Not pursuing my head fear(s) will not guarantee that I will be safe. ⊳

_____

_____

_____

⊲ Now say that aloud and believe it because it's true. ⊳

⊲ Are you willing to change how you look at fear and risk since there are no guarantees of either comfort or safety? Why or why not? ⊳

_____

_____

_____

♡ Do you agree that you might as well pursue those things that are head fears even if you have to do them afraid? Why or why not? ♡

_____

_____

_____

♡ Are you willing to look at your head fears about your deepest hopes and desires as a road map to the life you most want? Why or why not? ♡

_____

_____

_____

Wild *AND* Free

·» Step 2C: Prioritize «·

♡ Start with your answers on pages 271–272 (what/where you most want). Rewrite that list, ranking them by how much they matter to you from the most important to the least important. ♡

_____

_____

_____

_____

_____

_____

_____

_____

_____

_____

_____

_____

_____

_____

♡ Cross off anything that is a hope/desire belonging to someone else
that you somehow felt obligated to add to your own list. ♡

·» Step 2D: Define your deepest hopes and desires by tailoring them to fit only you «·

♡ Now for each item that's not crossed off on your prioritized list from page 274, customize it by adding as many specific details as possible so that you get what you most want. ♡

_____

_____

_____

_____

_____

_____

_____

_____

_____

_____

_____

_____

_____

_____

♡ More space to tailor what/where you most want. ♡

❧ More space to tailor what/where you most want. ❧

_____

_____

_____

_____

_____

_____

_____

_____

_____

_____

_____

_____

_____

❧ Read through your tailored list. ❧

❧ For each, answer this:
Does this hope and desire fit me like a second skin, excite me at the thought of it, represent the real me? ❧

❧ If the answer is yes, great. If the answer is no,
either add more specifics until you can answer with an honest yes or cross it off your list. ❧

·» Step 2E: Write them down «·

♡ A space to cleanly rewrite a list of tailored wants if you'd like or to doodle if you don't. ♡

_____

_____

_____

_____

_____

_____

_____

_____

_____

_____

_____

_____

_____

_____

♡ More space to cleanly rewrite a list of tailored wants if you'd like or to doodle if you don't. ♡

_____

_____

_____

_____

_____

_____

_____

_____

_____

_____

_____

_____

_____

_____

_____

_____

♡ More space to cleanly rewrite a list of tailored wants if you'd like or to doodle if you don't. ♡

_____

_____

_____

_____

_____

_____

_____

_____

_____

_____

_____

_____

_____

♡ A written list will increase your odds of success. ♡
♡ Reread this list daily even if you just scan it. ♡
♡ Use this list as a roadmap to get you to where you most want to go. ♡

·» Step 2F: Keep it to yourself «·

♡ Are you willing to keep your deepest hopes and desires to yourself even if you're excited about them? Why or why not? ♡

_____

_____

_____

♡ How will you feel and react if you share your deepest hopes and desires with someone and they don't respond the way you hope they will? ♡

_____

_____

_____

♡ Be sure to know this ahead of time and choose to share accordingly so you don't abandon yourself and abuse food or some other behavior/substance. ♡

·» Step Three «·
·» Imagine your ideal life «·

♡ Are you willing to believe that by simply thinking you can guide your weight-loss efforts and/or your efforts to stop abusing food? Why or why not? ♡

_____

_____

_____

৩ Are you willing to actively and daily imagine your ideal life? Why or why not? ৩

_____

_____

_____

৩ Write this: Overcoming food abuse is not all I envision for my ideal life. ৩

_____

_____

৩ Remember: your life has so much more to offer than just your weight and what you choose to eat. ৩

·» Step 3A: Say yes «·

৩ Write this: I say yes to my ideal life. ৩

_____

_____

৩ If you say no at any point, your journey down that particular path ends until you say yes again. ৩

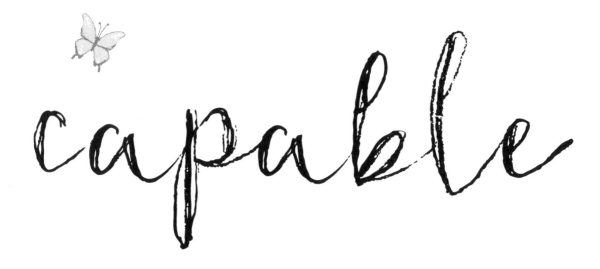

·» Step 3B: Begin with your hopes and desires «·

♡ Start with your answers on pages 274-280 (list of deepest hopes and desires). Close your eyes and picture your ideal life in your mind, incorporating those hopes and desires, as if you were right in the middle of it. Now write down what you envisioned using the present tense. Be specific with the details. Add images if you like. ♡

_____

_____

_____

_____

_____

_____

_____

_____

_____

_____

_____

_____

_____

♡ More space to envision your ideal life. ♡

_____

_____

_____

_____

_____

_____

_____

_____

_____

_____

_____

_____

_____

_____

_____

_____

♡ More space to envision your ideal life. ♡

_____

_____

_____

_____

_____

_____

_____

_____

_____

_____

_____

_____

_____

_____

_____

_____

·» Step 3C: Add in your gifts, talents, and passions «·

❧ Start with your answers on pages 283–285 (envisioning your ideal life). In relation to reaching that ideal life, what are your strengths? ☙

_____

_____

_____

_____

_____

_____

_____

❧ So you're going to empower yourself and emphasize those. ☙

❧ In relation to reaching that ideal life, what are your weaknesses? ☙

_____

_____

_____

_____

_____

_____

❧ So you know what not to emphasize nor spend a lot of your time on. ☙

In relation to reaching that ideal life, where is it necessary for you to strengthen your weaknesses?

_____

_____

_____

_____

_____

_____

_____

In relation to reaching that ideal life, where is it necessary for you to let go of your weaknesses and ask for help and/or delegate?

_____

_____

_____

_____

_____

_____

Yes, you're going to need some help from others to reach your ideal life; nobody can do it all.

·» Step 3D: Change the story you tell yourself «·

❍ Pick one of your deepest hopes or desires (from pages 283-285), preferably the one you're most drawn to doing. Write what bad things you believe could come to pass and the worst possible outcome you can think of if you pursued that hope/desire all the way to its end. ❧

_____

_____

_____

_____

_____

❍ Take a deep breath. ❧

❍ Now write the most amazing things that could come to pass in your life and the best possible outcome you can think of if you pursued that hope/desire all the way to its end. ❧

_____

_____

_____

_____

_____

❍ Take a deep breath. ❧

☙ Are you willing to stop telling yourself that worst-possible-outcome story and start telling yourself that best-possible-outcome story instead? Why or why not? ☙

_____

_____

_____

☙ Know this: the worst or best outcome is the story that you're telling yourself. ☙
☙ You will believe (and so live out) whatever story you tell yourself over and over. ☙

·» Step 3E: Keep your focus «·

☙ Are you willing to keep your ideal life as your focus? Why or why not? ☙

_____

_____

_____

☙ Focus will prevent you from winding up on detours that don't get you to where you most want to be. ☙

·» Step 3F: Keep your ideal life to yourself for now «·

☙ Are you willing to trust yourself and believe that your ideal life is solely about you and what you want to see come to pass? Why or why not? ☙

_____

_____

_____

☙ Be cautious when sharing your ideal life with others so you don't get derailed. ☙
☙ No need for anyone else's input or approval. ☙

·» Step Four «·
·» *Make an unbreakable promise to yourself* «·

◁ Are you willing to make an unbreakable promise to yourself that you are fully all-in? Why or why not? ▷

_____

_____

_____

◁ Are you willing to go as far as it takes to save your own life? Why or why not? ▷

_____

_____

_____

·» Step 4A: Turn your deepest hopes and desires into doable steps «·

◁ Write your best possible outcome from page 288 on the top line. Then write (in broad terms) all the steps/actions you can think of that you'll have to take to get yourself from where you are now to that best outcome. ▷

_____

_____

_____

_____

_____

♡ Space to write the actions you need to take to get to that best possible outcome. ♡

_____

_____

_____

_____

_____

_____

_____

_____

_____

_____

_____

_____

_____

_____

_____

_____

_____

_____

❧ Space to write the actions you need to take to get to that best possible outcome. ☙

_____

_____

_____

_____

_____

_____

_____

_____

_____

_____

_____

_____

_____

_____

_____

❧ Repeat for every hope/desire on pages 278–280 (or pages 274–277 if you didn't rewrite them).
Write the hope/desire, then the best possible outcome, then all the actions (in broad terms)
you'll have to take to get from where you are now to that best outcome. ☙

☙ Space to write a hope/desire, the best possible outcome, and actions to get there. ❧

_____

_____

_____

_____

_____

_____

_____

_____

_____

_____

_____

_____

_____

_____

_____

_____

◁ Space to write a hope/desire, the best possible outcome, and actions to get there. ▷

_____

_____

_____

_____

_____

_____

_____

_____

_____

_____

_____

_____

_____

_____

_____

_____

_____

♡ Space to write a hope/desire, the best possible outcome, and actions to get there. ♡

_____

_____

_____

_____

_____

_____

_____

_____

_____

_____

_____

_____

_____

_____

_____

_____

♡ Space to write a hope/desire, the best possible outcome, and actions to get there. ♡

_____

_____

_____

_____

_____

_____

_____

_____

_____

_____

_____

_____

_____

_____

_____

_____

·» Step 4B: Check your motivation, always «·

◇ Read through your list of doable steps on pages 290-296 . Then answer this: Are these all about you and what you want for your life? ◇

Yes   No

◇ Will achieving these steps give you self-fulfillment and personal satisfaction? ◇

Yes   No

◇ Will achieving these steps make you feel like you're having a successful life? ◇

Yes   No

◇ If the answer is no to any of those questions, then that particular doable step needs to be adjusted/rewritten so it will give you those things or you need to go back and cross it off your list. ◇

·» Step 4C: Let that doable-step list help you prioritize «·

◇ Are you willing to lighten your load and delegate to someone else? Why or why not? ◇

_____

_____

_____

◇ For each action on pages 290-296, circle/highlight anything that can be delegated to someone else. ◇

Step 4D: Answer probing questions honestly ⟪·

⟨ Be completely honest. ⟩

⟨ Are you willing to believe in your own worth and value no matter what? If not, why not? ⟩

_____

_____

⟨ Are willing to decide right now that reaching your ideal life matters deeply to you and that's reason enough to strive for it? If not, why not? ⟩

_____

_____

⟨ Are willing to believe you are strong, courageous, tenacious, intelligent, and fully capable of doing whatever needs to be done so you can have a life you love? If not, why not? ⟩

_____

_____

⟨ Are you willing to learn and experience new things? If not, why not? ⟩

_____

_____

⟨ Are you willing to stick with it even if it takes a long time (longer than you ever imagined it could)? If not, why not? ⟩

_____

_____

❧ Are you willing to spend time, money, energy, resources, or whatever it takes on yourself to facilitate your own growth and healing? If not, why not? ☙

_____

_____

❧ Are you willing to leave your comfort zone? If not, why not? ☙

_____

_____

❧ Are you willing to be open to growth and healing even if it's painful and/or requires you to do things that scare you? If not, why not? ☙

_____

_____

❧ Are you willing to face whatever obstacles/challenges arise? Or carry on even through setbacks? Or do whatever it is you need to do to thrive and flourish? If not, why not? ☙

_____

_____

_____

_____

❧ Are you willing to tell yourself the whole truth and also face the whole truth? If not, why not? ☙

_____

_____

ᴏ Are you willing to let go of everything that doesn't serve you so that you can become who you want and are meant to be? If not, why not? ᴏ

_____

_____

·» Step 4E: Count the costs of change «·
ᴏ Be completely honest. ᴏ

ᴏ Are you willing to sacrifice your time? If not, why not? ᴏ

_____

_____

ᴏ Are you willing to sacrifice your money? If not, why not? ᴏ

_____

_____

ᴏ Are you willing to sacrifice your current lifestyle? If not, why not? ᴏ

_____

_____

ᴏ Are you willing to sacrifice your social activities? If not, why not? ᴏ

_____

_____

_____

❧ Are you willing to sacrifice your family and/or other significant relationships? If not, why not? ❧

_____

_____

_____

❧ Are you willing to sacrifice whatever is necessary for your growth and healing? If not, why not? ❧

_____

_____

❧ Space to count any other costs to the best of your ability. ❧

_____

_____

_____

_____

_____

_____

_____

_____

_____

» Step 4F: Get rid of any escape clause «

⊲ Are you all-in no matter what? ⊳ _____

⊲ If your answer is yes, write this: I am fully all-in. I will reach my ideal life. Period. ⊳

_____

_____

_____

⊲ This is your unbreakable promise to yourself. ⊳

⊲ If your answer is no, answer these: Why don't you want to be all-in? What are you afraid will happen if you commit to your own best health and well-being? ⊳

_____

_____

_____

_____

_____

_____

_____

⊲ You won't succeed in reaching your ideal life if you have an escape clause. ⊳
⊲ So choose, right now, to be all-in and remove any kind of escape clause from your life. ⊳

·» Step 4G: Respect yourself «·

♡ Are you willing to always trust yourself and treat yourself with respect? If not, why not? ♡

_____

_____

_____

♡ Will you press on even if no one approves of your decisions/choices? If not, why not? ♡

_____

_____

_____

♡ Will you keep going even if no one else gives their stamp of approval to your ideal life? If not, why not? ♡

_____

_____

_____

♡ Will you carry on if there is no permission other than your own? If not, why not? ♡

_____

_____

_____

·» Step 4H: Honor yourself «·

♡ Are you willing to always have integrity with yourself? Why or why not? ♡

_____

_____

_____

♡ Write this: I am making this unbreakable promise to myself and no one else. ♡

_____

_____

♡ Write this: I am fully all-in. I promise to start and not procrastinate. I will carry on through whatever life brings my way. I will finish to see what I started through all the way to the end. I will reach my ideal life. Period. I will achieve what matters to me. ♡
♡ Then sign your name and date. ♡

_____

_____

_____

_____

_____

_____

Name:_____**Date:**_____

♡ So honor yourself and keep your word to yourself. ♡
♡ This is a longer version of your unbreakable promise to yourself. ♡

Step 4I: Choose to persevere «·

◌ Are you willing to persevere if you don't see immediate results, results in the time frame you had in mind, and/or results you weren't expecting? If not, why not? ◌

_____

_____

_____

◌ Will you persist in the direction of your ideal life and persevere until you reach a life that is true to you? Why or why not? ◌

_____

_____

_____

·» Step 4J: Be willing to grow slowly «·

◌ Are you willing to cultivate and practice patience every day? Why or why not? ◌

_____

_____

_____

◌ Are you willing to grow slowly, even if you don't like it? Why or why not? ◌

_____

_____

_____

✑ Go to pages 302 and 304. Write this and add it to your unbreakable promise:
I may go slowly, but I won't stop. ✑

·» Step 4K: Be hopeful «·

✑ Are you willing to hang on to hope no matter what? Why or why not? ✑

_____

_____

_____

✑ If you keep taking action and moving forward, you will get to your ideal life. Oh yes, you will. ✑

·» Step Five «·
·» Design your tiny targets «·

✑ Are you willing to take steps daily to reach your ideal life and keep every unbreakable promise you make to yourself? Why or why not? ✑

_____

_____

_____

✑ Are you willing to stop wishing, discussing, dreaming, etc. and instead take action toward your ideal life? Why or why not? ✑

_____

_____

_____

৶ Are you willing to accept that you, and you alone, are fully responsible for whether or not you reach your ideal life? Why or why not? ৽

_____

_____

_____

৶ Remember: there's only one life you can truly save in this world and that's your own. ৽

·» Step 5A: Say yes «·

৶ Are you willing to say yes and keep saying yes to moving in the direction of your ideal life? Why or why not? ৽

_____

_____

_____

৶ If you say no, your journey down that particular path ends. ৽

৶ If you say yes, write this three times: I say yes. ৽

_____

_____

_____

·» Step 5B: Create your tiny targets «·

♡ Begin with your doable step list, starting on page 290. Take just the first step you wrote. Write down all the smaller steps/actions you will have to take to reach the end result of just that first step. Make each step small enough that the thought of completing it doesn't scare you or at least scares you much, much less. Then repeat for all the other doable steps you wrote. ♡

♡ More space to create your tiny targets. ♡

_____

_____

_____

_____

_____

_____

_____

_____

_____

_____

_____

_____

_____

_____

_____

_____

♡ More space to create your tiny targets. ♡

_____

_____

_____

_____

_____

_____

_____

_____

_____

_____

_____

_____

_____

_____

_____

_____

_____

⊲ More space to create your tiny targets. ⊳

_____

_____

_____

_____

_____

_____

_____

_____

_____

_____

_____

_____

_____

_____

_____

♡ More space to create your tiny targets. ♡

_____

_____

_____

_____

_____

_____

_____

_____

_____

_____

_____

_____

_____

_____

_____

♡ More space to create your tiny targets. ♡

_____

_____

_____

_____

_____

_____

_____

_____

_____

_____

_____

_____

_____

_____

_____

_____

_____

·» Step 5C: Create specific tiny targets «·

♡ For each tiny target on pages 308–313, go back and add any specific details you'd like to hone that target so you get exactly what you want. Or you can use the space below to add more details. Add as many or as few details as you like. ♡

_____

_____

_____

_____

_____

_____

_____

_____

_____

_____

_____

_____

_____

_____

_____

♥ More space to create your specific tiny targets. ♥

_____

_____

_____

_____

_____

_____

_____

_____

_____

_____

_____

_____

_____

_____

_____

_____

_____

❧ More space to create your specific tiny targets. ☙

_____

_____

_____

_____

_____

_____

_____

_____

_____

_____

_____

_____

_____

_____

_____

❧ You will learn things as you grow and know yourself better. ☙

❧ Revisit your tiny target list to add or subtract specific details as you move forward toward your ideal life. ☙

·» Step 5D: Recognize your successes «·

♡ Write a list of the progress you're making, the successes you're having (no matter how big or small), and how far you've come. ♡

_____

_____

_____

_____

_____

_____

_____

_____

_____

·» Step 5E: Let that tiny target list guide all your actions and decisions «·

♡ Are you willing to refer back to your tiny target list when making decisions? If not, why not? ♡

_____

_____

♡ When faced with a choice/decision, ask this: Does this choice help me get to my ideal life or hinder me from getting to my ideal life? Then act accordingly. ♡

·» Step 5F: Define measurable progress for yourself «·

⊲ For each of your tiny targets, pick a measurement that works for you and write it down here. ⊳

_____

_____

_____

_____

_____

_____

_____

_____

_____

_____

_____

_____

_____

⊲ No one is policing you. You are defining and making progress because doing so matters deeply to you. ⊳

» Step 5G: Give yourself deadlines «

For each of your tiny targets, pick a deadline (date or time) that works for you, that both pushes/motivates you and is also realistic and achievable.

No one is policing you. Deadlines are for you and you alone to help you to keep going and to help you measure your progress. You're doing all this to save your own life.

·» Step 5H: Don't share your tiny targets with the public «·

↪ Answer these honestly: What will happen if someone gives you a snarky little comment about your tiny target? Will you use those comments as fuel and keep going? Or will you take them personally and give up? ↩

_____

_____

_____

_____

↪ If you feel like you need some support, look back to page 98 at the list of people you trust and tell only that person/group. ↩

·» Step 5I: Take action «·

↪ Are you willing to commit to taking action, one tiny target after the next after the next until you reach your ideal life? Why or why not? ↩

_____

_____

_____

↪ Taking action is the only way you will realize your ideal life. ↩

determined

·» Step 5J: Celebrate and reward yourself «·

⊘ Write a list of rewards you'd really like to receive. Now assign each of those rewards to a tiny target. ⊳

_____

_____

_____

_____

_____

_____

_____

_____

_____

_____

_____

_____

_____

⊘ Give yourself a reward every single time you reach a tiny target. Yes. Every. Single. Time. ⊳

·» Step Six «·
·» Create your lifework «·

� All of us exchange our time on this earth for something. Wouldn't you rather exchange your time for working toward and achieving your ideal life? If not, why not? ◦

_____

_____

_____

◦ Are you willing to make reaching your ideal life your focus? Why or why not? ◦

_____

_____

_____

◦ Are you willing to make your gifts, talents, and passions your purpose for being alive? Why or why not? ◦

_____

_____

_____

◦ Are you ready and willing to be responsible for your own life and how it turns out? Why or why not? ◦

_____

_____

_____

↻ Are you ready and willing to let your lifework act like an anchor during the stormy times of your life? Why or why not? ↺

_____

_____

_____

·» Step 6A: Combine Your Ideal Life And Unbreakable Promise With Your Tiny Targets«·

↻ Read through your answers from Imagine Your Ideal Life (starting on page 281), Make An Unbreakable Promise To Yourself (starting on page 290), and Design Your Tiny Targets (starting on page 306). ↺

↻ Mark those pages and revisit them often, preferably daily. ↺

↻ Let your lifework become your focus, know which tiny target you need to hit each day, see your progress. ↺

·» Step 6B: Decide your lifework is both vital to you and a necessity for your happiness «·

↻ Do you believe that your lifework needs to be accomplished by you in order for you to feel like you are having a successful life? Why or why not? ↺

_____

_____

_____

↻ Are you willing to be your sole motivation and disregard what anyone else says/ thinks/does about your lifework? Why or why not? ↺

_____

_____

↻ Remember: this is your life you're working to save. ↺

Are you willing to see your lifework as a necessity in your life for your own happiness? Why or why not?

_____

_____

_____

Step 6C: Take action

Are you willing to do the next tiny target on your list every day until you reach your ideal life? Why or why not?

_____

_____

_____

Train your brain and make a habit out of forward progress.

Step 6D: Celebrate and reward yourself

Are you willing to have integrity with yourself and give yourself a reward every single time you reach a tiny target? Why or why not?

_____

_____

_____

Giving yourself rewards will also reinforce for you the importance of your lifework.

·» Step 6E: Assess and monitor your progress «·

Write a list of all your victories and successes (no matter how big or small).

_____

_____

_____

_____

_____

_____

_____

_____

_____

_____

Answer this: Are you on track, making progress and meeting your deadlines? If not, what changes do you need to make?

_____

_____

_____

_____

_____

❧ Are you growing and moving forward? If not, what do you need to address so you can grow and move forward? ☙

_____

_____

_____

_____

❧ Are you productive (getting things finished) or just busy (lots of work but nothing completed)? ☙

_____

_____

❧ Are you stalled? If so, why? ☙

_____

_____

_____

_____

_____

_____

_____

♡ Are you making excuses? If so, why? ♡

_____

_____

_____

_____

_____

_____

_____

♡ Are you afraid? (If so, how can you make your tiny target(s) smaller? ♡

_____

_____

_____

_____

_____

_____

_____

☙ Are you willing to make yourself accountable and keep an honest eye on how you're doing? Why or why not? ❧

_____

_____

_____

·» Step 6F: Cut yourself some slack «·

☙ Are you willing to believe there is only success or learning? Why or why not? ❧

_____

_____

_____

☙ Are you willing to practice self-compassion, being kind, gentle, and patient with yourself always? Why or why not? ❧

_____

_____

_____

☙ Remember: you can always just start again right where you are. ❧

gifted

·» Step 6G: Remember you're on a journey «·

♡ Write this: I hereby give myself permission to bring myself happiness as I work my way from one tiny target to the next. ♡

♡ Then sign your name and date. ♡

_____

_____

_____

_____

Name:_____Date:_____

♡ So honor yourself and keep your word to yourself. ♡

·» Step 6H: Let your lifework fuel you «·

♡ Are you willing to look at your lifework as a source of encouragement, motivation, inspiration, and joy in your life? Why or why not? ♡

_____

_____

_____

♡ Are you willing to let your lifework befriend you, pulling you upward and forward? Why or why not? ♡

_____

_____

_____

·» Step 6l: Finish «·

⊘ Are you willing to keep going until you have seen what you've started all the way through to the end and reach your ideal life? Why or why not? ⊳

_____

_____

_____

⊘ Remember: it doesn't matter in the least how slowly you go as long as you don't stop. ⊳

·» Step Seven «·
·» Live with purpose «·

⊘ Do you understand that you're choosing the life that you're living? If not, why not? ⊳

_____

_____

_____

⊘ To have a different life, you must make different choices. ⊳

⊘ Are you willing to say yes to head fears, regardless of how much they scare you, and say no to those people, places, and/or things that don't move you toward your ideal life? Why or why not? ⊳

_____

_____

_____

Are you willing to deeply believe that you're worth saving, that what you have to offer matters, and that you have something in your lifetime that needs to be completed by you? Why or why not?

_____

_____

_____

Do you believe you're on an urgent mission to complete your lifework? Why or why not? And if not, are you willing to believe it?

_____

_____

_____

Are you willing to let go of your history so you can move forward unencumbered? Why or why not?

_____

_____

_____

Are you willing to teach others and believe you're in collaboration with others, trying to help them realize their potential while you are busy realizing your own? Why or why not?

_____

_____

_____

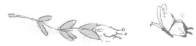

·» Step 7A: Coach yourself «·

♡ What reassuring words do you most need to hear right now? ♡

_____

_____

_____

_____

♡ What do you most need to have/do/say right now in this moment to help you reach your ideal life? ♡

_____

_____

_____

_____

♡ Give/do/say it to yourself right now. ♡

·» Step 7B: Always look for the open path «·

♡ Write a list of paths that you really want to go down that seem to be blocked to you. ♡

_____

_____

_____

_____

❧ More space for paths that seem to be blocked to you. ☙

_____

_____

_____

_____

_____

❧ What other paths are open to you that will still get you to where you want to be? ☙

_____

_____

_____

_____

_____

❧ What other choices do you have? ☙

_____

_____

_____

_____

_____

⊲ What other decisions do you need to make that will move you forward? ⊳

_____

_____

_____

_____

_____

⊲ What other actions can you take that will make you feel alive? ⊳

_____

_____

_____

_____

_____

⊲ Are you willing to let go of any blocked path(s)? Why or why not? ⊳

_____

_____

_____

⊲ Do yourself a kindness and stop wasting time that you cannot get back. ⊳
⊲ Find a way that's open to you and choose to go down that path instead. ⊳

·» Step 7C: Have an abundance mentality «·

ᴗ Write this: I believe that there's always enough for me. ᴗ

_____

_____

ᴗ Now say it aloud. ᴗ

ᴗ Write this: I believe there is enough to go around for everybody. ᴗ

_____

_____

ᴗ Now say it aloud. ᴗ

ᴗ Write this: I believe in more life for all. ᴗ

_____

_____

ᴗ Now say it aloud. ᴗ

ᴗ Write this: I believe I will always get everything I need and more. ᴗ

_____

_____

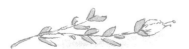
ᴗ Now say it aloud. ᴗ
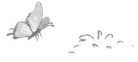

❧ Write five things you are grateful for in your life today. ❧

1. _____

2. _____

3. _____

4. _____

5. _____

❧ Repeat often. ❧

·» Step 7D: Take a leap of faith «·

❧ Are you willing to get out of your comfort zone, step into the unknown, and take the leap of faith no matter what? Why or why not? ❧

_____

_____

_____

❧ Your comfort zone will expand and grow with every step you take. ❧

❧ Are you willing to prove to yourself just how much courage you have? Why or why not? ❧

_____

_____

_____

❧ Take a leap of faith. You will amaze yourself at how much you are truly capable of. ❧

·» Step 7E: Change your focus «·

♡ Are you willing to take your focus off food and/or other substances/behaviors that you're abusing and put it squarely on reaching your ideal life? Why or why not? ♡

_____

_____

_____

·» Step 7F: Prioritize «·

♡ Are you willing to put yourself as number one on your daily to-do list? Why or why not? ♡

_____

_____

_____

♡ Are you willing to prioritize what's most important to you? Why or why not? ♡

_____

_____

_____

♡ You make the schedule you keep. ♡
♡ You also choose the people, places, things, and/or activities that will help you or hinder you. ♡

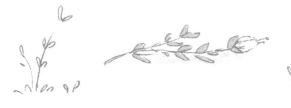

·» Step 7G: Surrender the outcome «·

⌁ Are you willing to let go of trying to control the outcome and instead relax into the process and the journey? Why or why not? ⌁

_____

_____

_____

⌁ Breathe your way through. ⌁

·» Step 7H: Be patient «·

⌁ Are you willing to accept that there's a reason you're not yet where you want to be? Why or why not? ⌁

_____

_____

_____

⌁ Be kind and gentle with yourself as you wait. ⌁

⌁ What lesson(s) can you find in whatever you're going through? ⌁

_____

_____

_____

_____

♡ More space to record lesson(s) you find in whatever you're going through. ♡

_____

_____

_____

_____

_____

·» Step 71: Remember you're still growing «·

♡ Are you willing to remain open every day? Why or why not? ♡

_____

_____

_____

♡ Are you willing to believe you still have time? If not, why not? ♡

_____

_____

_____

focused

·» Oh, some science (part one) «·

⊘ Are you willing to be congruent (expressing yourself and taking actions that are in line with what you believe)? Why or why not? ⊘

_____

_____

_____

⊘ Congruence will work to change your brain and, in turn, change your life. ⊘

·» Oh, some science (part two) «·

⊘ Write some strength to yourself (words you most need to hear right now) and add your name after each phrase. ⊘

_____

_____

_____

_____

_____

_____

_____

_____

_____

⊘ Now say all those phrases out loud. ⊘

·» Oh, some science (part three) «·

✎ Write a list of any more successes. ✎
✎ Add to your list from page 317. ✎

_____

_____

_____

_____

_____

_____

_____

_____

_____

_____

_____

_____

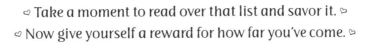

✎ Take a moment to read over that list and savor it. ✎
✎ Now give yourself a reward for how far you've come. ✎

·» **This is a practice and a process** «·

⊘ What worked for you during this chapter? What didn't? ⊘

_____

_____

_____

_____

_____

_____

⊘ Always, always, always find what works for you and do that. ⊘
⊘ You have permission to let go, right now, of anything that doesn't work for you. ⊘

⊘ Write a list of things you've learned from your mistakes. ⊘

_____

_____

_____

_____

_____

_____

⊘ Learn what you can, come at it again from a wiser perspective, then move on. ⊘
⊘ Remember: every mistake is simply a brand new chance to do it better the next time. ⊘

·» Notes or doodles «·

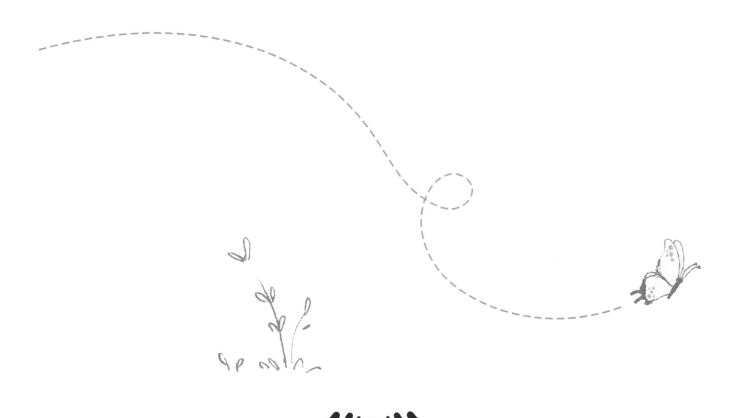

Chapter Seven!

·» The Hero's Journey «·

Do you want to be victorious on your own hero's journey? Why or why not?

_____

_____

_____

Are you willing to believe your life is your story and you can always make some edits and/or rewrite the ending? Why or why not?

_____

_____

_____

Considering your life is your story, what edits would you make and/or how would you rewrite the ending?

_____

_____

_____

_____

_____

·⟩⟩ **Stage One: The calling and saying no to it** ⟨⟨·

☙ What do you know/feel/believe the calling is on your life? ❧

_____

_____

_____

_____

_____

☙ Do you want to know what the calling is on your life? Why or why not? ❧

_____

_____

_____

☙ Have you said no to the calling on your life? If so, how and why? ❧

_____

_____

_____

_____

_____

◁ Do you agree that it's the refusal of the calling that leads you to abuse food? Why or why not? ▷

_____

_____

_____

◁ If you said no to the calling, are you willing to change your mind and accept the calling on your life right now? Why or why not? ▷

_____

_____

_____

◁ You can always say yes and start right where you are. ▷

·» Stage Two: Cosmic help «·

◁ Are you willing to fully commit to being the hero of your own story? If not, why not? ▷

_____

_____

_____

◁ Are you willing to be fully responsible for your efforts? Why or why not? ▷

_____

_____

_____

◁ Remember: no one is coming to fix it. ▷

❧ Write this: I truly and fully commit to being the hero of my own story. I will take action and produce results. I am on a mission and I will keep going until I achieve what I set out to do. ❧

❧ Then sign your name and date. ❧

_____

_____

_____

_____

_____

_____

Name:_____**Date:**_____

❧ So honor yourself and keep your word to yourself. ❧

❧ Are you willing to believe and trust that you'll get what you need right when you need it? Why or why not? ❧

_____

_____

_____

❧ Cosmic help comes to you once you truly and fully commit then believe and trust. ❧

·» Stage Three: Crossing into the unknown and a dark night of the soul «·

❧ Do you believe you're safe in your comfort zone? If so, why? ❧

_____

_____

_____

_____

❧ There is no sure thing, even in your comfort zone. ❧

❧ Are you willing to choose to be brave and courageous? Why or why not? ❧

_____

_____

_____

❧ If you don't believe you are brave, all you need to do is change your mind. ❧

❧ Are you willing to trust yourself? Why or why not? ❧

_____

_____

_____

❧ You are trustworthy and strong enough to handle whatever comes your way. ❧

❦ Are you willing to believe that in the end everything works out for your good to get you to where you're meant to be? Why or why not? ❧

_____

_____

_____

❦ Are you willing to be all-in? If not, why not? ❧

_____

_____

_____

❦ Are you willing to stop running away from your weaknesses? Why or why not? ❧

_____

_____

_____

❦ What will you choose: fight it out and become someone new or go back to your old self and perish? Why? ❧

_____

_____

_____

◁ Are you willing to believe your gifts, talents, passions, and purpose were given to you to share for a greater good? Why or why not? ▷

_____

_____

_____

◁ Do you believe who you're meant to be serves a larger whole? Why or why not? ▷

_____

_____

_____

◁ Have you ever called on divine or supernatural help? If so, when and why? If not, are you willing to if needed? ▷

_____

_____

_____

◁ Are you willing to be fully responsible for taking action and fixing your own life? Why or why not? ▷

_____

_____

_____

◁ All you have to do is keep moving toward the life that you want to have and refuse to stop. ▷

☙ Are you willing to be open to the possibility that your life can be so much greater than you envisioned? Why or why not? ❧

_____

_____

_____

☙ Are you willing to let go of who you thought you would be so you can become who you're meant to be? Why or why not? ❧

_____

_____

_____

·» Stage Four: Trials, tribulations, and temptation's trap «·

☙ Have you already been hit with some obstacles, challenges, and/or tests? If so, what were they? ❧

_____

_____

_____

_____

_____

_____

_____

၁ Are you willing to keep going when you get hit with obstacles, challenges, and/or tests? Why or why not? ၁

_____

_____

_____

၁ Some kind of adversity is inevitable. ၁

၁ Do you believe defeat is always optional? Why or why not? ၁

_____

_____

_____

၁ Write this three times: Food will not fix it. ၁

1. _____

2. _____

3. _____

၁ Do you believe you are capable of fixing it? Why or why not? ၁

_____

_____

_____

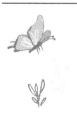

၁ One small step (tiny, if need be) at a time, you can. Oh yes, you can. ၁
၁ Just keep saying yes, taking action, and moving forward, and you will. ၁

◌ What have your trials and tribulations already taught you? ◌

_____

_____

_____

_____

_____

_____

◌ Are you willing to let trials and tribulations teach you? Why or why not? ◌

_____

_____

_____

◌ Find out just how strong, courageous, tenacious, intelligent, persevering that you are. ◌

◌ What do you do when you're faced with failure? ◌

_____

_____

_____

_____

_____

◌ The answer matters. The answer is your character. ◌

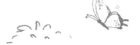

ᘒ What kind of person do you want to be? ᘒ

_____

_____

_____

_____

_____

_____

_____

ᘒ That's the question that the trials and tribulations will ask and the one that you'll have to answer. ᘒ

ᘒ Write a list of instances where you have been tempted to pause, veer off in another direction, and/or quit altogether. ᘒ

_____

_____

_____

_____

_____

_____

_____

◌ Of those instances, which ones did you say yes and give in to? ◌

_____

_____

_____

_____

_____

◌ Remember: if you choose the temptation, your quest ends. ◌
◌ You can always change your mind and say no. ◌

◌ Of those instances, which ones did you push through and say no to? ◌

_____

_____

_____

_____

_____

_____

 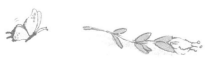 ◌ Celebrate your victories! ◌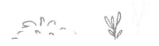

♡ If you are currently in temptation's trap, are you willing to abandon the temptation? If not, why not? ♡

_____

_____

_____

♡ Are you willing to choose, right now, to say no when temptation comes your way? Why or why not? ♡

_____

_____

_____

♡ Are you willing to look temptation in the eye, holler no, and keep carrying on with what you know you need to do to get to where you most want to be? Are you willing to do that over and over? Why or why not? ♡

_____

_____

_____

·» Stage Five: Experiencing unconditional love and the restoration of the power balance «·

♡ Do you believe you are worthy of experiencing unconditional love? Why or why not? ♡

_____

_____

⤫ Are you willing to experience unconditional love? Why or why not? ⤫

_____

_____

_____

⤫ Will you choose to befriend yourself, completely trust yourself, and give yourself unconditional love through whatever may come your way? Why or why not? ⤫

_____

_____

_____

⤫ Are you willing to take responsibility for your own happiness and how you treat yourself in the good times and the bad? Why or why not? ⤫

_____

_____

_____

⤫ Do you believe that the Universe is a supportive, nurturing, friendly place? Why or why not? If not, are you willing to consider the possibility that it is? ⤫

_____

_____

_____

❧ Write this 3 times: I believe the Universe is a friendly place that wants to see me succeed. ☙

1. _____

2. _____

3. _____

❧ Now repeat daily for 66 days. ☙

❧ Are you willing to combine trusting and befriending yourself with believing the Universe is a friendly place? Why or why not? ☙

_____

_____

_____

❧ Write a list of who or what you believe holds all the power over you and that you feel powerless against. ☙

_____

_____

_____

_____

_____

_____

_____

❧ Refer back to Chapter Five (the vampires, starting on page 204) if needed. ☙

❧ Why do you choose to stay with people/places/things that diminish you? ☙

_____

_____

_____

_____

_____

_____

_____

_____

_____

_____

❧ You don't have to make that same choice anymore. ☙
❧ You can choose differently, starting right now. ☙

❧ Are you willing to confront and then defeat whoever or whatever you believe holds the ultimate power over you? Why or why not? ☙

_____

_____

_____

❧ You won't be able to be the hero in your own life until you do. ☙

↩ What steps do you need to take to rid yourself of those things that make you feel powerless? ↪

_____

_____

_____

_____

↩ Refer back to Chapter Five (the vampires, starting on page 204) if needed. ↪
↩ Do those steps for yourself and take your power back. ↪

·» Stage Six: Death to self «·

↩ Write a list of people/places/things that you let go of that also felt like a little death (something over forever) to you. ↪

_____

_____

_____

_____

_____

_____

_____

_____

_____

☙ Are you willing and ready to stop clinging and let go of everything that no longer serves you? Why or why not? ☙

_____

_____

_____

☙ Are you willing and ready to stop fighting against yourself? Why or why not? ☙

_____

_____

_____

☙ Are you willing and ready to choose never to go back to living the way you were before and to being the person you were before? Why or why not? ☙

_____

_____

_____

☙ Are you willing and ready to let go of who you used to be and what you thought you would be so that you can become who you are meant to be? Why or why not? ☙

_____

_____

_____

⋄ Write a list of your little callings. ⋄

_____

_____

_____

_____

_____

_____

_____

_____

⋄ Now write the word yes next to each one. ⋄

⋄ Are you willing and ready to move forward, with confidence and trust in yourself, in the direction you know you need to go? Why or why not? ⋄

_____

_____

_____

trustworthy

·» Stage Seven: Goal achieved «·

⊲ Write a list of numbers/goals/targets you were aiming for that you reached. ⊳

_____

_____

_____

_____

_____

_____

_____

_____

⊲ Celebrate your victories! ⊳

⊲ Are you willing and ready to break free and move on a forward and straight trajectory in your life? Why or why not? ⊳

_____

_____

_____

❧ Are you willing and ready to no longer live in fear of food or in shame about yourself? Why or why not? ❧

_____

_____

_____

❧ Are you willing and ready to have food no longer be your focus? Why or why not? ❧

_____

_____

_____

❧ Are you willing and ready to have what you actually want to have/be/do/say with your life become your focus instead? Why or why not? ❧

_____

_____

_____

❧ Are you willing and ready to blaze your own path, the path that you were actually meant to be on, a path that matters to you? Why or why not? ❧

_____

_____

_____

·» Stage Eight: Not wanting to come back, making a careful return, and some guidance for the return «·

♡ Write a list of hard things in your life that were in some way a gift to you. ♡

_____

_____

_____

_____

_____

_____

_____

_____

♡ What lesson(s) did you learn from those hard things you went through. ♡

_____

_____

_____

_____

_____

_____

_____

⊲ Are you willing to pass on that wisdom to others? Why or why not? ⊳

_____

_____

_____

⊲ Which will you choose: hang out in paradise by yourself OR open yourself up and invite others into your life? Why? ⊳

_____

_____

_____

_____

_____

_____

⊲ Are you willing to experience a deeper way of being in the world than you ever experienced before? Why or why not? ⊳

_____

_____

_____

⊲ You'll probably be scared to share what you've learned. That's okay. Choose to do it anyway. ⊳

❤ What, if anything, scares you about the return to your life as the new you? ❤

_____

_____

_____

_____

_____

_____

_____

_____

❤ Are you ready to share your newfound knowledge? Why or why not? ❤

_____

_____

_____

❤ Are you willing to treat this step with the seriousness it deserves? Why or why not? ❤

_____

_____

_____

❧ Are you willing to wait to share your newfound knowledge until you're secure in yourself and your ability to handle life as it comes? Why or why not? ❧

_____

_____

_____

❧ Are you willing to trust yourself to know when it's time to share your wisdom? Why or why not? ❧

_____

_____

_____

❧ Write this: I give myself permission to keep my newfound knowledge to myself until I'm prepared for whatever may get thrown at me. ❧
❧ Then sign your name and date. ❧

_____

_____

_____

_____

Name:_____**Date:**_____

❧ Just be sure not to drag out your return because of fear. ❧
❧ You'll know when you're ready. ❧

෪ Do you want to return to your normal life? Why or why not? ෫

_____

_____

_____

෪ Are you willing to let others help you integrate as you return to your normal life (and not in a come-fix-it or do-it-for-you way)? Why or why not? ෫

_____

_____

_____

෪ Write a list of people who have helped you along your way. ෫

_____

_____

_____

_____

_____

_____

_____

_____

෪ Now be grateful for them and thank them. ෫

◁ Write what you need. ▷

_____

_____

_____

_____

_____

◁ Now ask someone you trust to help you get what you need. ▷
◁ Keep moving forward. ▷

◁ Are you willing to be open to whatever form the guidance for the return will take? Why or why not? ▷

_____

_____

_____

◁ Just don't ever fall into the mindset of looking for someone to come fix it and/or do it for you. ▷

·» Stage Nine: Returning from the unknown «·

◁ Have you dismissed/discarded this step in the past (achieved your goal then not put into practice everything you've learned)? If so, when, why, and what was the end result? ▷

_____

_____

_____

♡ Use this space to give yourself credit and bask in your achievement. ♡

_____

_____

_____

♡ Do you believe your efforts are over once you reach your goal? Why or why not? ♡

_____

_____

_____

♡ Are you willing to remember and put into daily practice everything you learned? Why or why not? ♡

_____

_____

_____

♡ Are you willing to keep taking action and moving forward in your life? Why or why not? ♡

_____

_____

_____

↵ Write this: I commit to not going back to who I once was and to the way I did things before. ↩

↵ Then sign your name and date. ↩

_____

_____

_____

Name:_____**Date:**_____

↵ Now honor and respect yourself by keeping your word to yourself. ↩

↵ Are you willing to teach what you've learned to others? Why or why not? ↩

_____

_____

_____

↵ What's the best way for you to teach what you've learned to others? ↩

_____

_____

_____

↵ Help both yourself and others by passing on your wisdom. ↩

worthwhile

·» Stage Ten: Finding balance and freeing yourself «·

᷄ Are you ready and willing to be comfortable and at ease with yourself, with who you are as a person, and to move through your life with confidence and determination? Why or why not? ᷅

_____

_____

_____

᷄ Do you fully understand that inner peace starts from within? Why or why not? ᷅

_____

_____

_____

᷄ Are you ready and willing to stop fighting yourself and to cease letting head fear stop you? Why or why not? ᷅

_____

_____

_____

᷄ Are you ready and willing to heal the rift/hole inside yourself caused by incongruence and take action to move forward in the direction you know you need to go? Why or why not? ᷅

_____

_____

_____

Are you ready and willing to believe that:
- all things really do work out for your good
- life is rigged in your favor
- you are supported wherever you may go
- you will get everything you need right when you need it
- no matter what is happening in your life, no matter how hard it might be to go through, everything is going to be okay
- you are both strong enough and capable enough to handle anything that comes your way
- the only place you can change anything is in the present moment
- your life isn't about impressing anyone but is about becoming who you are meant to be
- creating a life that deeply matters to you is what will make you finally feel fulfilled
- the only life you can truly save is your own

If not, why not?

_____

_____

_____

_____

_____

_____

_____

_____

_____

_____

_____

❧ What death(s) (in whatever form that death takes) do you fear? ☙

_____

_____

_____

_____

_____

_____

_____

_____

❧ Are you ready and willing to lose your fear of death (in whatever form that death takes)? Why or why not? ☙

_____

_____

_____

❧ Are you ready and willing to let things that aren't serving you anymore fall away? Why or why not? ☙

_____

_____

_____

⊘ Are you ready and willing to change and grow and do whatever you like with your life to become the person you most want to be? Why or why not? ಬ

_____

_____

_____

⊘ Are you ready and willing to free yourself from the confines and limitations of fear? Why or why not? ಬ

_____

_____

_____

⊘ Are you ready and willing to relax into your life and take life as it comes because you're strong enough to handle anything that gets thrown at you? Why or why not? ಬ

_____

_____

_____

⊘ Are you ready and willing to start where you are and trust that all of life really is aimed at helping you grow into the person that you are meant to be? Why or why not? ಬ

_____

_____

_____

·» This is a practice and a process «·

⊘ What worked for you during this chapter? What didn't? ⊘

_____

_____

_____

_____

_____

_____

_____

⊘ Always, always, always find what works for you and do that. ⊘
⊘ You have permission to let go, right now, of anything that doesn't work for you. ⊘

⊘ Write a list of things you've learned from your mistakes. ⊘

_____

_____

_____

_____

_____

⊘ Learn what you can, come at it again from a wiser perspective, then move on. ⊘
⊘ Remember: every mistake is simply a brand new chance to do it better the next time. ⊘

Epilogue!

·» Yes, you are going to have to change «·
♡ You can put off going into a chrysalis. ♡

♡ Have you put off your transformation? If so, how? ♡

_____

_____

_____

♡ Are you ready and willing to say yes and let the transformation of yourself and your life happen? Why or why not? ♡

_____

_____

_____

♡ You have to go through the struggle. ♡

♡ What are you struggling with right now? ♡

_____

_____

_____

❧ Are you ready and willing to believe that whatever you're struggling with right now is just to help strengthen you for the good things about to come your way? Why or why not? ❧

_____

_____

_____

❧ Are you ready and willing to keep going through the struggle, all the way until you make it through to the other side? Why or why not? ❧

_____

_____

_____

❧ Have you looked to others to do the work for you? If so, how? ❧

_____

_____

_____

❧ Are you ready and willing to stop looking for others to do the work for you and instead do the work yourself? Why or why not? ❧

_____

_____

_____

❧ You can't rush your transformation. ☙

❧ Have you tried to rush your transformation? If so, how? ☙

_____

_____

_____

_____

❧ Are you ready and willing to cultivate patience and not rush your transformation? Why or why not? ☙

_____

_____

_____

❧ Write this: I commit to letting my transformation happen naturally. I commit to practicing patience and not rushing my transformation. ☙
❧ Then sign your name and date. ☙

_____

_____

_____

_____

Name:_____**Date:**_____
❧ Now honor and respect yourself by keeping your word to yourself. ☙

☙ The only way you can get your wings and fly is to transform. ❧

☙ Are you ready and willing to let go of the old you and how you used to do things, and instead make changes to your life that will help you grow and transform into the person you're meant to become? Why or why not? ❧

_____

_____

_____

☙ Once you transform, you can never go back to the way you were before. ❧

☙ Are you ready and willing to spread your metaphorical wings, trusting this is what you were made to do, and fly? Why or why not? ❧

_____

_____

_____

☙ What will you choose: no to the life before you then try to fit yourself back inside the life that once held you OR yes to the life before you and let go and trust that you'll rise to become who you want and are meant to be? Why? ❧

_____

_____

_____

_____

·»· A few reminders ·«·

◌ Are you ready and willing to make you and only you the reason you want to be thinner and/or you want to stop abusing food? Why or why not? ◌

_____

_____

_____

◌ You are reason enough and worth the effort. ◌

◌ Do you harbor a sprig of hope that being thin equals your life being perfect or at least a lot closer to perfection than it is now? Why or why not? ◌

_____

_____

_____

◌ Are you ready and willing to believe that being thin will not fix all your problems? Why or why not? ◌

_____

_____

_____

◌ Are you ready and willing to believe that being thinner makes you a healthier person, not a better person? Why or why not? ◌

_____

_____

_____

❧ Are you ready and willing to understand your weight may fluctuate and that's okay? Why or why not? ☙

_____

_____

_____

❧ What weight/size do you feel your best? ☙

_____

_____

❧ What weight-fluctuation-number boundaries do you want to set? ☙

_____

_____

❧ Write a list of things you have to offer. ☙

_____

_____

_____

_____

_____

_____

❧ You are so much more than just a number on a scale. ☙

Are you ready and willing to accept that you're on a journey for the whole of your life, so no need to hurry? Why or why not?

_____

_____

_____

Are you ready and willing to not go running back to the way(s) you used to do things, hoping that maybe, just maybe, it'll work this time? Why or why not?

_____

_____

_____

Are you ready and willing to find what works for you because you've got your whole life to figure it out? Why or why not?

_____

_____

_____

Have you bragged about your weight loss and/or no longer abusing food, especially to get praise/admiration/etc.? If so, how?

_____

_____

_____

_____

꙳ Have you ever believed, once you reached your goal weight, that you can go back to abusing food and/or eating whenever you want? If so, when and how did that turn out for you? ꙳

_____

_____

_____

_____

꙳ Are you ready and willing to stay humble? Why or why not? ꙳

_____

_____

_____

꙳ Are you ready and willing to not care what anyone else thinks about your weight loss and/or cessation of abusing food? Why or why not? ꙳

_____

_____

_____

꙳ How many times have you tried to lose weight and/or stop abusing food? How long have you been at it? ꙳

꙳ See your answer on page 21 for how long you've been on the diet-go-round. ꙳

_____

_____

꙳ None of that matters. ꙳
꙳ The only thing that matters is that you keep trying until you find what works for you. ꙳

৶ Are you ready and willing to believe that you only fail if you quit? Why or why not? ৸

_____

_____

_____

৶ It truly doesn't matter how slowly you go as long as you don't stop. ৸

৶ Are you ready and willing to carry on and make some adjustments and figure out what you're doing wrong? Why or why not? ৸

_____

_____

_____

৶ Are you ready and willing to let patience be your friend? Why or why not? ৸

_____

_____

_____

৶ Are you ready and willing to believe that you can and will overcome whatever gets thrown at you, one (tiny, if need be) step at a time? Why or why not? ৸

_____

_____

_____

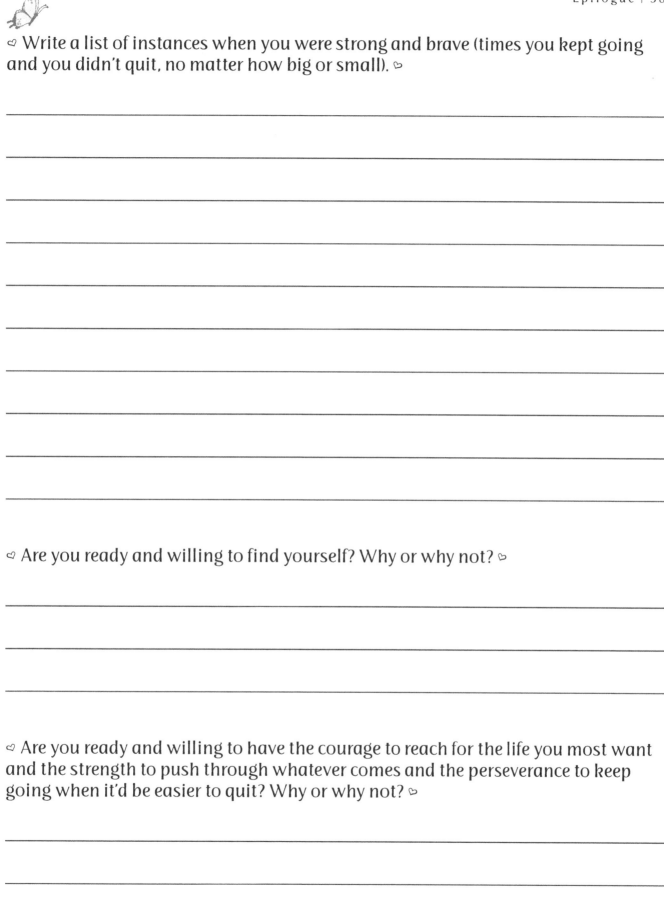

◁ Write a list of instances when you were strong and brave (times you kept going and you didn't quit, no matter how big or small). ▷

◁ Are you ready and willing to find yourself? Why or why not? ▷

◁ Are you ready and willing to have the courage to reach for the life you most want and the strength to push through whatever comes and the perseverance to keep going when it'd be easier to quit? Why or why not? ▷

·» A note on cherry picking «·

♡ Are you ready and willing to give yourself permission to cherry pick from all the information you've gotten so you can create a life for yourself that you love by doing those things that work best for you? Why or why not? ♡

_____

_____

_____

♡ Remember: at the end of each chapter, you wrote what worked for you and what didn't. ♡
♡ Let those answers be your guide. ♡

♡ Are you ready and willing to abandon any rigid food rules and instead always listen to your body and let it be your guide? Why or why not? ♡

_____

_____

_____

♡ Are you ready and willing to ask yourself in a kind voice—What's the matter? What do you need?—in those moments when you want to abuse food? Why or why not? ♡

_____

_____

_____

⊘ Are you ready and willing to honor your answers and give yourself what you need? Why or why not? ⊳

⊘ Are you ready and willing to give yourself permission, right now and always, to create a plan that works for you and also to change that plan whenever you need to? Why or why not? ⊳

·» This is a practice and a process «·

⊘ What worked for you during this chapter? What didn't? ⊳

⊘ Always, always, always find what works for you and do that. ⊳

⊘ You have permission to let go, right now, of anything that doesn't work for you. ⊳

❧ Write a list of things you've learned from your mistakes. ☙

_____

_____

_____

_____

_____

_____

_____

❧ Learn what you can, come at it again from a wiser perspective, then move on. ☙
❧ Remember: every mistake is simply a brand new chance to do it better the next time. ☙

❧ Are you ready and willing to strive for progress and do the best you can? Why or why not? ☙

_____

_____

_____

❧ Are you ready and willing to show yourself compassion instead of tearing yourself down? Why or why not? ☙

_____

_____

_____

♡ Are you ready and willing to not give up on yourself, to just take a deep breath and start again, right where you are? Why or why not? ♡

_____

_____

_____

♡ You can always (always, always) change your mind at any point. ♡
♡ You can always (always, always) start again right where you are. ♡

♡ Are you ready and willing to go create a life you love? Why or why not? ♡

_____

_____

_____

♡ Go be happy. ♡
♡ Go create a life you love. ♡

I'm possible

·» A page to write what you're grateful for if you want «·
♡ Or to doodle if you don't. ♡

» A page to write what you're grateful for if you want «
⌃ Or to doodle if you don't. ⌃

·» A page to chart your weight if you want «·
⸫ Or to doodle if you don't. ⸫

trust

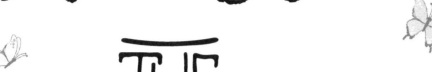

THE

journey

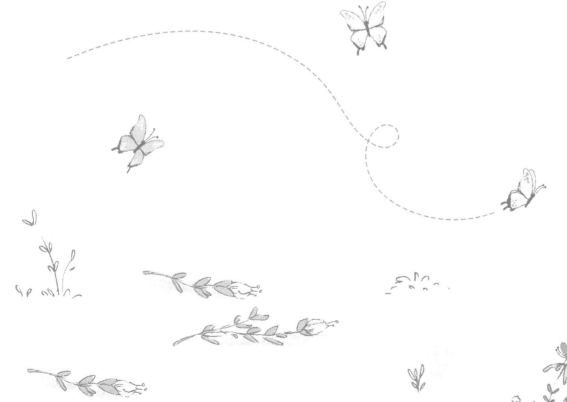

·›› Disclosures and Disclaimers ‹‹·

This book is published in print format. All trademarks and service marks are the properties of their respective owners. All references to these properties are made solely for editorial purposes. Except for marks actually owned by the Author or the Publisher, no commercial claims are made to their use, and neither the Author nor the Publisher is affiliated with such marks in any way.

Unless otherwise expressly noted, none of the individuals or business entities mentioned herein has endorsed the contents of this book.

Limits of Liability & Disclaimers of Warranties

Because this book is a general educational information product, it is not a substitute for professional advice on the topics discussed in it.

The materials in this book are provided "as is" and without warranties of any kind either express or implied. The Author and the Publisher disclaim all warranties, express or implied, including, but not limited to, implied warranties of merchantability and fitness for a particular purpose. The Author and the Publisher do not warrant that defects will be corrected. The Author does not warrant or make any representations regarding the use or the results of the use of the materials in this book in terms of their correctness, accuracy, reliability, or otherwise. Applicable law may not allow the exclusion of implied warranties, so the above exclusion may not apply to you.

Under no circumstances, including, but not limited to, negligence, shall the Author or the Publisher be liable for any special or consequential damages that result from the use of, or the inability to use this book, even if the Author, the Publisher, or an authorized representative has been advised of the possibility of such damages. Applicable law may not allow the limitation or exclusion of liability or incidental or consequential damages, so the above limitation or exclusion may not apply to you. In no event shall the Author or Publisher total liability to you for all damages, losses, and causes of action (whether in contract, tort, including but not limited to, negligence or otherwise) exceed the amount paid by you, if any, for this book.

You agree to hold the Author and the Publisher of this book, principals, agents, affiliates, and employees harmless from any and all liability for all claims for damages due to injuries, including attorney fees and costs, incurred by you or caused to third parties by you, arising out of the products, services, and activities discussed in this book, excepting only claims for gross negligence or intentional tort.

You agree that any and all claims for gross negligence or intentional tort shall be settled solely by confidential binding arbitration per the American Arbitration Association's commercial arbitration rules. Your claim cannot be aggregated with third party claims. All arbitration must occur in the municipality where the Author's principal place of business is located. Arbitration fees and costs shall be split equally, and you are solely responsible for your own lawyer fees.

Facts and information are believed to be accurate at the time they were placed in this book. All data provided in this book is to be used for information purposes only. The information contained within is not intended to provide specific legal, financial, tax, physical or mental health advice, or any other advice whatsoever, for any individual or company and should not be relied upon in that regard. The services described are only offered in jurisdictions where they may be legally offered. Information provided is not all-inclusive, and is limited to information that is made available and such information should not be relied upon as all-inclusive or accurate.

For more information about this policy, please contact the Author at the website address listed in the Copyright Notice at the front of this book.

IF YOU DO NOT AGREE WITH THESE TERMS AND EXPRESS CONDITIONS, DO NOT READ THIS BOOK. YOUR USE OF THIS BOOK, INCLUDING PRODUCTS, SERVICES, AND ANY PARTICIPATION IN ACTIVITIES MENTIONED IN THIS BOOK, MEAN THAT YOU ARE AGREEING TO BE LEGALLY BOUND BY THESE TERMS.

Affiliate Compensation & Material Connections Disclosure

This book may contain references to websites and information created and maintained by other individuals and organizations. The Author and the Publisher do not control or guarantee the accuracy, completeness, relevance, or timeliness of any information or privacy policies posted on these websites.

You should assume that all references to products and services in this book are made because material connections exist between the Author or Publisher and the providers of the mentioned products and services ("Provider"). You should also assume that all website links within this book are affiliate links for (a) the Author, (b) the Publisher, or (c) someone else who is an affiliate for the mentioned products and services (individually and collectively, the "Affiliate").

The Affiliate recommends products and services in this book based in part on a good faith belief that the purchase of such products or services will help readers in general.

The Affiliate has this good faith belief because (a) the Affiliate has tried the product or service mentioned prior to recommending it or (b) the Affiliate has researched the reputation of the Provider and has made the decision to recommend the Provider's products or services based on the Provider's history of providing these or other products or services.

The representations made by the Affiliate about products and services reflect the Affiliate's honest opinion based upon the facts known to the Affiliate at the time this book was published.

Because there is a material connection between the Affiliate and Providers of products or services mentioned in this book, you should always assume that the Affiliate may be biased because of the Affiliate's relationship with a Provider and/or because the Affiliate has received or will receive something of value from a Provider.

Perform your own due diligence before purchasing a product or service mentioned in this book.

The type of compensation received by the Affiliate may vary. In some instances, the Affiliate may receive complimentary products (such as a review copy), services, or money from a Provider prior to mentioning the Provider's products or services in this book.

In addition, the Affiliate may receive a monetary commission or non-monetary compensation when you take action by using a website link within in this book. This includes, but is not limited to, when you purchase a product or service from a Provider after going to a website link contained in this book.

Health Disclaimers

As an express condition to reading to this book, you understand and agree to the following terms.

This book is a general educational health-related information product. This book does not contain medical advice.

The book's content is not a substitute for direct, personal, professional medical care and diagnosis. None of the exercises or treatments (including products and services) mentioned in this book should be performed or otherwise used without prior approval from your physician or other qualified professional health care provider.

There may be risks associated with participating in activities or using products and services mentioned in this book for people in poor health or with pre-existing physical or mental health conditions.

Because these risks exist, you will not use such products or participate in such activities if you are in poor health or have a pre-existing mental or physical condition. If you choose to participate in these risks, you do so of your own free will and accord, knowingly and voluntarily assuming all risks associated with such activities.

Earnings & Income Disclaimers

No Earnings Projections, Promises or Representations
For purposes of these disclaimers, the term "Author" refers individually and collectively to the author of this book and to the affiliate (if any) whose affiliate hyperlinks are referenced in this book.

You recognize and agree that the Author and the Publisher have made no implications, warranties, promises, suggestions, projections, representations or guarantees whatsoever to you about future prospects or earnings, or that you will earn any money, with respect to your purchase of this book, and that the Author and the Publisher have not authorized any such projection, promise, or representation by others.

Any earnings or income statements, or any earnings or income examples, are only estimates of what you might earn. There is no assurance you will do as well as stated in any examples. If you rely upon any figures provided, you must accept the entire risk of not doing as well as the information provided. This applies whether the earnings or income examples are monetary in nature or pertain to advertising credits which may be earned (whether such credits are convertible to cash or not).

There is no assurance that any prior successes or past results as to earnings or income (whether monetary or advertising credits, whether convertible to cash or not) will apply, nor can any prior successes be used, as an indication of your future success or results from any of the information, content, or strategies. Any and all claims or representations as to income or earnings (whether monetary or advertising credits, whether convertible to cash or not) are not to be considered as "average earnings".

Testimonials & Examples
Testimonials and examples in this book are exceptional results, do not reflect the typical purchaser's experience, do not apply to the average person and are not intended to represent or guarantee that anyone will achieve the same or similar results. Where specific income or earnings (whether monetary or advertising credits, whether convertible to cash or not), figures are used and attributed to a specific individual or business, that individual or business has earned that amount. There is no assurance that you will do as well using the same information or strategies. If you rely on the specific income or earnings figures used, you must accept all the risk of not doing as well. The described experiences are atypical. Your financial results are likely to differ from those described in the testimonials.

The Economy
The economy, where you do business, on a national and even worldwide scale, creates additional uncertainty and economic risk. An economic recession or depression might negatively affect your results.

Your Success or Lack of It
Your success in using the information or strategies provided in this book depends on a variety of factors. The Author and the Publisher have no way of knowing how well you will do because they do not know you, your background, your work ethic, your dedication, your motivation, your desire, or your business skills or practices. Therefore, neither the Author nor the Publisher guarantees or implies that you will get rich, that you will do as well, or that you will have any earnings (whether monetary or advertising credits, whether convertible to cash or not), at all.

Businesses and earnings derived therefrom involve unknown risks and are not suitable for everyone. You may not rely on any information presented in this book or otherwise provided by the Author or the Publisher, unless you do so with the knowledge and understanding that you can experience significant losses (including, but not limited to, the loss of any monies paid to purchase this book and/or any monies spent setting up, operating, and/or marketing your business activities, and further, that you may have no earnings at all (whether monetary or advertising credits, whether convertible to cash or not).

Forward-Looking Statements
Materials in this book may contain information that includes or is based upon forward-looking statements within the meaning of the Securities Litigation Reform Act of 1995. Forward-looking statements give the Author's expectations or forecasts of future events. You can identify these statements by the fact that they do not relate strictly to historical or current facts. They use words such as "anticipate," "estimate," "expect," "project," "intend," "plan," "believe," and other words and terms of similar meaning in connection with a description of potential earnings or financial performance.

Any and all forward looking statements here or on any materials in this book are intended to express an opinion of earnings potential. Many factors will be important in determining your actual results and no guarantees are made that you will achieve results similar to the Author or anybody else. In fact, no guarantees are made that you will achieve any results from applying the Author's ideas, strategies, and tactics found in this book.

Purchase Price

Although the Publisher believes the price is fair for the value that you receive, you understand and agree that the purchase price for this book has been arbitrarily set by the Publisher or the vendor who sold you this book. This price bears no relationship to objective standards.

Due Diligence

You are advised to do your own due diligence when it comes to making any decisions. Use caution and seek the advice of qualified professionals before acting upon the contents of this book or any other information. You shall not consider any examples, documents, or other content in this book or otherwise provided by the Author or Publisher to be the equivalent of professional advice.

The Author and the Publisher assume no responsibility for any losses or damages resulting from your use of any link, information, or opportunity contained in this book or within any other information disclosed by the Author or the Publisher in any form whatsoever.

YOU SHOULD ALWAYS CONDUCT YOUR OWN INVESTIGATION (PERFORM DUE DILIGENCE)
BEFORE BUYING PRODUCTS OR SERVICES FROM ANYONE. THIS INCLUDES PRODUCTS AND SERVICES
SOLD VIA WEBSITE LINKS REFERENCED IN THIS BOOK.

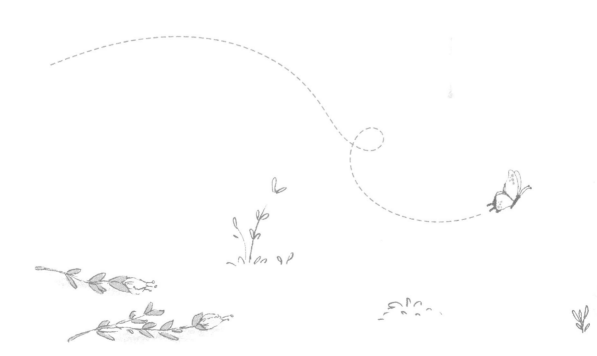

CPSIA information can be obtained
at www.ICGtesting.com
Printed in the USA
LVHW101103201219
641163LV00004B/6/P